# THE
# BRITISH
# SCHOOLS
# OF
# PSYCHOANALYSIS

## THE LIBRARY OF CLINICAL PSYCHOANALYSIS

### A SERIES OF BOOKS EDITED BY
### STEVEN J. ELLMAN

This series is intended to show the depth, flexibility and vigor of contemporary Freudian thought. It is by no means a series that can be equated with classical psychoanalysis or ego psychology, but rather we intend to show how contemporary Freudians are able to meaningfully integrate a variety of positions into the scaffolding of Freudian tenets. Goldman's and especially Bach's work show the richness and depth that can be achieved within such a framework.

Freud's Technique Papers:
   A Contemporary Perspective
      *Steven J. Ellman*

In Search of the Real:
   The Origins and Originality
   of D. W. Winnicott
      *Dodi Goldman*

In One's Bones:
   The Clinical Genius of
   Winnicott
      *Dodi Goldman, Editor*

The Language of Perversion
   and the Language of Love
      *Sheldon Bach*

The British Schools
   of Psychoanalysis:
   Pluralism and Convergence
   in the Clinical Setting
      *Daniel Hill and Carole Grand,
      Editors*

# THE BRITISH SCHOOLS OF PSYCHOANALYSIS

## Pluralism and Convergence in the Clinical Setting

ANALYSTS IN SESSION
Contemporary Freudian
Independent
Modern Kleinian

COMMENTARY
(*Americans*)
Steven Ellman
Fred Pine
Robert Wallerstein

(*British*)
Marion Burgner
Michael Parsons
John Steiner

Edited by:
Daniel Hill, Ph.D., and Carole Grand, Ph.D.

JASON ARONSON INC.
*Northvale, New Jersey*
*London*

This book was set in 11 pt. Baskerville by Alpha Graphics of Pittsfield, New Hampshire and printed and bound by Book-mart Press of North Bergen, New Jersey.

**Library of Congress Cataloging-in-Publication Data**

The British schools of psychoanalysis / pluralism and convergence
  in the clinical setting  / edited by Daniel Hill & Carole Grand.
      p.  cm.
  Includes bibliographical references and index.
  ISBN 1-56821-745-5
  1. Psychoanalysis—History.  2. Pluralism.  3. British Psycho-
Analytical Society.  I. Hill, Daniel.  II. Grand, Carole.
BF173.P644  1996
150.19'5—dc20                                        95-32112

Manufactured in the United States of America. Jason Aronson Inc. offers books and cassettes. For information and catalog write to Jason Aronson Inc., 230 Livingston Street, Northvale, New Jersey 07647.

We dedicate this book to our spouses,

Donna Bassin and Stanley Grand.

# About the Editors

Daniel Hill, Ph.D., began his professional life as an educator—co-founder of the New London Free School, high school teacher, school psychologist, and principal at the Walden School in New York City. Trained as an analyst at the New York University's Postdoctoral Program in Psychoanalysis, he is on the faculties of the New Hope Guild Child and Adolescent Training Program and The Contemporary Center for Advanced Psychoanalytic Studies. He is also an associate editor of *Psychoanalytic Inquiry* and a member of the editorial board of *Psychoanalysis and Psychotherapy*. Dr. Hill is the founder of the Committee for the Development of Online Services at the NYU Postdoctoral Program and the founder and director of PsyBC, an educationally oriented service producing programs for mental health professionals on the Internet. He is also in private practice in NYC.

Carole Grand, Ph.D., received her psychoanalytic training at New York University's Postdoctoral Program in Psychotherapy and Psychoanalysis. She is a member of the Institute for Psychoanalytic Training and Research and the International Psychoanalytical Association. Dr. Grand teaches and supervises in the New Hope Guild Child and Adolescent Psychoanalytic Psychotherapy Training Program and in its Continuing Adult Psychotherapy Program. She is also a member of its Board of Directors. She is faculty member and supervisor in the Child and Adolescent Program at the Post Graduate Center for Mental Health and on the faculty of the Metropolitan Institute for Training in Psychoanalytic Psychotherapy.

Dr. Grand was trained first in child and adolescent psychotherapy before she received her adult psychoanalytic training at NYU. She maintains a private practice in Manhattan in psychoanalysis and psychotherapy with children, adolescents, and adults.

# Contents

## III Commentary: American Analysts

## IV Commentary: British Analysts

## V Synthesis and Conclusion

# Preface

There have been three major influences determining the make-up of this study. The earliest was the concern that psychoanalysts rarely see, close up, the clinical work of senior analysts. We see the process notes of supervisees and we hear about how our own supervisors think, but the likelihood is that the only senior analyst we ever see in practice is our own. Although this is a fine learning experience, it is hardly a representative sample. In 1988, we began a series of workshops at the New York University Postdoctoral Program in which senior analysts presented process notes from a single session along with a running commentary of their thoughts during the session and their reasons for making the interventions they did. We called the series "Analysts in Session." The idea was to bring the work of senior analysts, their clinical-life-as-lived, into the educational domain. We believe these workshops provided us with another source of learning to refine the tools of our trade.

A second influence was Robert Wallerstein's generative work on psychoanalytic pluralism. He articulated a tension in the psychoanalytic world in which several schools of psychoanalysis, all claiming truth, vie for attention and power. Underlying the tension is a set of problems that involve theoretical, social, and political issues. In this book we are interested in the theoretical issues inherent in the problems of pluralism and, more specifically, with the relationship between theories and theories-as-practiced. We wanted to look at the differences and similarities between theories, not as they are espoused in books and articles but as they are practiced in the consulting room.

Finally, a third influence was the idea that psychoanalytic pluralism is a driving problem for psychoanalysis. We believe that the pluralism that "plagues" psychoanalysis is a healthy problem, that it reflects the growth of the field, and that, like adolescence, it is difficult to live with but crucial for maturity. We wanted to use pluralism to drive forward the development of psychoanalytic theory.

These three aims—educational, theoretical, and progressive—are at the heart of this book. To accomplish our goals, we decided to look at the British Psycho-Analytical Society. We chose this group first because it has a remarkable group of senior analysts who have trained under many of our most respected and original theorists. These theorists (e.g., Balint, Fairbairn, Anna Freud, Guntrip, Klein, and Winnicott) have made far-reaching contributions to what is now a world-wide pluralism. Second, it has a documented history that reveals the development and effects of that pluralism. And finally, American psychoanalysis has become less insular and has increasingly turned its attention toward the British Society asking, "What can we learn from their experience and from their changing understanding of mental life?"

Our aims required a carefully planned format—a design for a study. A group was formed of presenters and commentators. The presenters were training analysts chosen from among the three groups of the British Psycho-Analytical Society: one Contemporary Freudian, one Modern Kleinian, and one Independent. The Contemporary Freudian analyst and the Modern Kleinian analyst were women. The Independent analyst was a man. Each presenter provided process notes from a single session in which oedipal material was prominent and also provided a running commentary about their interventions and thoughts during the session.

Although we believed that the status of the oedipal conflict could use re-examination, the request for a session with oedipal material was based mainly on pragmatic concerns. That is, we needed a common moment that would anchor the comparisons of metapsychologies to a discussion of theories-as-practiced and that would juxtapose the data with regard to content as well as process.

Our next concern was with the commentary. We decided to use two groups of three commentators. The first group is composed of three American psychoanalysts who are interested in the issue of pluralism per se, each with a distinct point of view. The second group of commentators is from the British Society, one from each of the groups that constitute it. They were chosen in part to serve as a check on the representativeness of the presenters in relation to the groups with which they are affiliated and in part to bring their own perspectives to bear on the sessions presented. The commentators were asked to compare and contrast the theories-as-practiced when faced with oedipal material.

Finally, we have set ourselves the task of summarizing and integrating the commentary, synthesizing it when possible, and occasionally commenting on it.

## A Note about Confidentiality

The presenters have taken care to protect the identities of their patients by altering the material. As a further precaution, we have decided not to use the names of the three British presenters. Instead, they are referred to as the Freudian analyst, the Kleinian analyst, and the Independent analyst. The full names of two of these groups in the British Psycho-Analytical Society are the Contemporary Freudian Group and the Modern Kleinian Group. To make it less cumbersome for the reader, we have dropped the words "Contemporary" and "Modern."

Daniel Hill
Carole Grand

# Acknowledgments

We are reminded that the Director of NYU's Post Doctoral Program, Bernie Kalinkowitz, was still very much with us in 1988 when we first conceived the "Analysts in Session" workshops. He attended, along with his wife Teddy, all seventeen of them. Always the educator and a promoter of a heterogeneous atmosphere, Bernie supported and encouraged us to continue to organize new workshops each year, and finally the conference that has led to the end product, this book. So, along with our appreciation to the Freudian Colloquium Committee and the Freudian faculty of the Post Doctoral Program in Psychotherapy and Psychoanalysis, under whose auspices we developed the "Analysts in Session" series, we are indebted to Bernie Kalinkowitz.

On a more personal note, we want to thank our respective spouses, Donna Bassin and Stanley Grand, for their exceptional forbearance, frequent wise counsel, and unflagging belief in the value of our project. We are also grateful to the Bassin-Hill children, Ari and Ezra, who complained only mildly about losing time with their father so that he could confer (once again) on the telephone.

We appreciate those commentators who took time off from their busy schedules to read other parts of this book and write words of encouragement: Fred Pine, Robert Wallerstein, and Marion Burgner.

Without Steve Ellman's original suggestion that we pub-
lish with Jason Aronson, we might not have a finished product to talk about and, certainly, without his help, this book
may have been born nameless.

We would be remiss if we did not mention the wisdom
and level-headedness of Jason Aronson and Michael Moskowitz
who managed to steer us through some troubled waters along
the way to publication without drowning, and Judy Cohen,
whose fine editing turned a tiresome job into a pleasure.

We wish also to acknowledge the thoughtfulness, creativity, and critical insight that each of our six commentators,
both British and American, have contributed to the mortar
of this work and out of which we were able to draw our comparisons, come to our conclusions, and generally build this
book.

Finally, it is to our British presenters who generously
shared their clinical work with us, first at NYU and then in
this book, that we are most indebted, for without them, this
project would have ended prematurely.

Daniel Hill and Carole Grand

# Contributors

**Marion Burgner**  Training and Child Analyst, British Psycho-Analytical Society; Faculty, Anna Freud Centre.

**Steven Ellman**  Professor of Clinical Psychology, City University of New York; Training and Supervising Analyst, President (1994–1996), Institute for Psychoanalytic Training and Research; Clinical Professor, New York University Post-Doctoral Program in Psychoanalysis and Psychotherapy.

**Carole Grand**  New York University PostDoctoral Program in Psychoanalysis and Psychotherapy; Member, Institute for Psychoanalytic Training and Research; Board of Directors, Faculty and Supervisor, New Hope Guild Child and Adolescent Therapy Training Program.

**Daniel Hill**  New York University PostDoctoral Program in Psychoanalysis and Psychotherapy; Faculty and Supervisor, The Contemporary Center for Advanced Psychoanalytic Studies; Faculty, New Hope Guild Child and Adolescent Therapy Training Program.

**Michael Parsons**  Training Analyst, British Psycho-Analytical Society; Member, International Psychoanalytical Association.

**Fred Pine**  Professor, Albert Einstein College of Medicine; Clinical Professor, New York University PostDoctoral Pro-

gram in Psychoanalysis and Psychotherapy; Training and
Supervising Analyst, New York Freudian Society.

**John Steiner**   Training Analyst,  British Psycho-Analytical
Society; Consultant Psychotherapist, Tavistock Clinic.

**Robert Wallerstein**   Emeritus Professor of Psychiatry, University of California, San Francisco School of Medicine; Training and Supervising Analyst, San Francisco Psychoanalytic
Institute; Past President, American Psychoanalytic Association; Past President, International Psychoanalytical Association.

**The Freudian Analyst**   Training Analyst, The British Psycho-
Analytical Society.

**The Independent Analyst**   Training Analyst, The British
Psycho-Analytical Society.

**The Kleinian Analyst**   Training Analyst, The British Psycho-
Analytical Society.

# I

# INTRODUCTIONS TO THE STUDY

# 1

# Pluralism as a Driving Force in Psychoanalysis

*DANIEL HILL*

Robert Wallerstein (1990), in his plenary address to the International Psychoanalytical Association, surveyed the international practice of psychoanalysis and established psychoanalytic plurality as a central problem for exploration. He asked whether we have "one psychoanalysis or many" and concluded that we have both. In our clinical work he finds common ground and one psychoanalysis. In our metapsychologies he sees many. This does not disturb him because he views our metapsychologies as metaphors we cling to in our struggles to ply our dangerous trade and to grasp what is beyond our reach. Of course, many disagree with the notion of a disjuncture between theory and technique, and many disagree with his notion of a clinical common ground. However, psychoanalytic diversity has become a *driving problem* for psychoanalysis, not only because of the dialectical tensions it evokes but also because the fact of incompatible theories operating as truths is a constant reminder that psychoanalytic theory is still not mature. In the past, Freud's original work, seen as incomplete here and wrong there, was still the pre-eminent stimulus to further thought. Now it is joined by pluralism as a ubiquitous impetus to development.

Our pluralism evokes other questions that complement the question of common ground. What are the sources of our diversity? What accounts for the divisiveness that has accompanied it? And more to the point of this study, what will come of it?

The sources of our diversity is a fascinating problem that will influence the next stage of development. Is it that the theories reflect the minds of the theorists? To what extent do history, culture, and language determine our theories? Are the different metapsychologies a function of presumptions of what is pathological and what is healthy? Do we choose theories that suit our personalities and shy away from the theories and techniques that make us uncomfortable in the clinical setup?

Along with an understanding of the sources of diversity, ecumenical projects and any effort toward theoretical integration will benefit from an understanding of why the diversity has been accompanied by divisiveness. For ultimately, the divisiveness interferes with explorations of the relevant issues—of the *validity* of each new set of ideas, of how one should test such a validity, and of how well our metapsychologies can accommodate those ideas that are valid.

In some ways the history of psychoanalytic ideas does not distinguish it from other intellectual disciplines. All are subject to vested interests. The fights among the partisans are no less painful, do equal damage to the development of ideas, and make life equally difficult for those entering the field. Yet, in important ways, psychoanalysis is different. From the beginning psychoanalysis took itself to be a movement, one that was revolutionary and under attack. From this initial conception developed a religiosity. Ironically, each of the schools that broke with tradition seems to have also fancied itself a movement, conducting *its* affairs with measures of "theoretical correctness" and allegiances to articles of faith. It is an atmosphere engendered by the scarcity of empirically testable hypotheses. Theory became dogma. Theorists became icons.

In thinking about how our divisiveness is different from that of other disciplines, it must also be noted that the various theories informed our personal analyses, were helpful to us or not, and gave us a stamp of approval in our professional subworlds. We have special identifications with our theories because they become our mirrors—mirrors that we guard religiously. Thus, along with the transferences and the political and economic motives to which all disciplines are subject, we are coping with the regressive processes that accompany a narcissism of difference. And where divisiveness is a problem, there will be struggles to overcome the impulses to reduce and dichotomize in the service of insulating oneself and excluding others.

It is perhaps this kind of narcissism that has blinded us to the fact that, for many of us, contingency was the primary factor determining which theoretical orientation informed our personal analyses and our training. Some such contingencies are the time and place where we entered the field, the discipline from which we migrated, our finances, and even our schedules.

Finally, if theoretical pluralism is inherently unstable for a discipline looking for truths, then what is to come of it? Fifteen years ago there were basic theoretical choices to be made that no longer seem so pressing—choices between a baby striving for differentiation and another striving for attachment, between a libido that was seeking pleasure and another that was seeking objects, between a theory of pathogenesis based in conflict and another based in deficit. In the heat of the moment—the transferences and politics of institutional life—it was hard to acknowledge that one had meager resources for making a genuine choice. Only recently has it become respectable to consider the ecumenical idea that it may not be necessary to make these choices—that they may have been false dichotomies. Times have changed, and the problem now seems to be, "What will be the framework for integration?" What will come out of pluralism is, of course, unclear. However, pluralism itself has become a catalyst for development.

The study was conducted through the auspices of the New York University Postdoctoral Program in Psychoanalysis and Psychotherapy (NYU Postdoc). NYU Postdoc is also where Dr. Grand and I were trained. Like the British Psycho-Analytical Society, it is a home to psychoanalytic diversity. Although founded to transcend the theoretical walls, the walls were imported. There are now four competing groups within the institute: Freudians, Independents, Interpersonalists, and Relationalists. For all the difficulties that come with this diversity, one is relatively free of insularity. When I have crossed the internal borders at NYU Postdoc I often am brought back to a statistical rule—that the variance within groups is always greater than the variance between groups. And increasingly have seen an overlap of accepted ideas.

Several assumptions guided the planning for the study. First we assumed that a convergence of some sort is taking place—that as the world grows smaller and as the interpenetration of ideas speeds up, psychoanalysts of whatever persuasion are forced into an integration of one kind or another. The study also is based on the assumption that the best route to that integration is through clinical data. Clinical theory may or may not be our common ground, clinical-theory-as-proposed may not be the same as practiced, and our metapsychologies may determine our perception of the data, but process notes are the closest thing we have to a bedrock upon which to build an integration. Metaphor or not, theory becomes real in clinical-life-as-lived.

The chapters that follow constitute a study of psychoanalytic pluralism. Moreover, this study uses that very pluralism to advance our understanding of the clinical process. In that regard and to the extent that the outcome has advanced the field, it is an instance of pluralism as a driving force in psychoanalysis—a microcosm reflecting its macrocosm.

## Reference

Wallerstein, R. S. (1990). Psychoanalysis: the common ground. *International Journal of Psycho-Analysis* 71:3–20.

# 2

# A Brief History
# of the British
# Psycho-Analytical Society

## *CAROLE GRAND*

Since our presenters are each affiliated with one of the three groups of the British Psycho-Analytical Society, a brief synopsis of the historic events that led to their formation will set the stage for the presentations and commentaries that follow. The events that took place from the 1920s to the mid-1940s in the psychoanalytic world in England embroiled our greatest thinkers in a tumultuous battle that was to shape the British Psycho-Analytical Society and provide all of us with thorny theoretical and technical issues to argue and debate long into the future. Riccardo Steiner (1985) points out that these events can be seen as just part of a series of clashes that have regularly punctuated the course of psychoanalysis since its birth. Psychoanalytic training in the United States is still reverberating from the clash between psychoanalytic lay groups in this country, the American Psychoanalytic Association and the International Psychoanalytical Association. We at N.Y.U. are very familiar with the intensity of feelings that can be generated by theoretical clashes that have the potential to tear down a divided house. We too have learned to live peaceably under one roof and have begun to be enriched by each other's presence. Books have been written about this historic period in the development of psychoanalytic thought.

In 1926, Melanie Klein settled permanently in Britain. She arrived at a time when her teachings seemed to be a natural outgrowth of the views held by many British psychoanalysts, who were not traditionally reverent to any overarching theory. They were open to new ideas and were already making use of direct observation of children and infants. English culture had a history of interest in children and the child's place in society and so was very interested in Klein's discoveries in child psychoanalysis. By the time the war began, and with the work of John Bowlby and Anna Freud, the early object relationship had already taken a prominent place in psychoanalytic thinking. The importance of pregenital factors in the development of the internal object relationship and perception of reality was recognized, and a new picture of psychoanalysis had begun to emerge.

In the early 1920s in Vienna, Anna Freud was developing her views on child analytic techniques. After a brief initial period in which Anna Freud praised Klein for discovering the use of the play technique for child psychoanalysis, it became clear that there were fundamental disagreements in the theoretical beliefs of the two women as well as in their approaches to technique. The following are some of the basic issues on which they differed: the dating of the oedipal complex to the second half of the first year of life, the early emergence of the ego and the superego, the emphasis on infantile phantasies and their phylogenetic heritage, the sadistic and hostile nature of the infant's superego and its relationship to infantile anxiety and guilt, the centrality of the death instinct or the destructive impulse, an object relationship based on projection and introjection, and the early use of drive and transference interpretations.

The implications of Klein's theories clashed with the classical Freudian position in fundamental ways. These theories diminished the importance of regression, disputed the concept of primary narcissism, rejected a compartmentalized theory of psychosexual stages with its implications for object relationships and character development, and raised many controversies about technique, one of which centered on the immediate and direct interpretation of both the negative and positive transference. By 1927, it was evident from the criticism of Anna Freud's book on child analytic technique by Klein and her supporters that there would be a polarization between London and Vienna. The bitter nature of the controversies that followed from the 1920s and continued throughout the 1930s threatened the very fabric of psychoanalytic training at the British Institute and life in the British Psycho-Analytical Society.

Freud tried to stay out of things but was pulled into the struggle by Anna in 1927 after she realized how harsh the criticism of her papers was. Particularly in his correspondence with Jones, he began to bring the full weight of his position into defense of her work and against the personal attacks on her as well.

Opposition to Klein's ideas became vehement in 1935 when Klein presented her paper, "A Contribution to the Psychogenesis of Manic–Depressive States." This paper introduced the concept of the depressive position that, for Klein, replaced the oedipal complex as the core problem and developmental achievement. When Anna Freud arrived in England with her father in 1939, Klein's views had already been challenged, and two groups had formed, each with its supporters and detractors. The rosters of the British Psycho-Analytical Society had swelled because of the war on the Continent, and this too was to influence the balance in the Society. Klein's supporter's at that time included Susan Isaacs, Sylvia Payne, Joan Riviere, Donald Winnicott, Paula Heimann, and Herbert Rosenfeld, among others. Today, we closely associate the names of Bion, Betty Joseph, and Hanna Segal with the Modern Kleinians.

In 1942, the dissension in the Society was intolerable.

Klein felt that she was not departing from the main concepts of Freudian theory and that she was in fact advancing Freud's theory. She believed that she was enriching Freudian theory with the addition of her two positions: her emphasis on aggression and her modifications of views on infantile affects and anxieties and female sexuality. In contrast, Anna Freud believed that Klein not only was moving up the timetable of human development and advocating technical modifications but that she was also challenging the underpinnings of Freudian metapsychology and describing a different model of the mind.

While all this was taking place, a middle group was emerging. This group was strongly influenced by the work of Winnicott and Bowlby and was not allied with either the Klein or the Anna Freud group. They did not form a school or training program of their own, but adhered to a more eclectic, developmental model based on observation and direct clinical work. The middle group, which from 1973 on became known as the Independent group, has as its main interests the nature of the patient–analyst relationship, an emphasis that it shares with the Kleinians and the Freudians; their respective subjective experiences; the object-relating and object-seeking infant; the influence of the real object relationship; and anxiety in separating from the first maternal object. Their conceptual formulations are deeply rooted in their clinical work. Winnicott's emphasis on the empathy of the analyst and his ability to provide a holding environment for the patient was a guiding principle of technique that allowed the patient to reveal his true self. Some of the names (in addition to Winnicott) we now associate with this group are Balint, Fairbairn, Bollas, Masud Khan, Margaret Little, and Nina Coltart, to name a few. Not all have remained in the British Psycho-Analytical Society.

By 1942, the battle had become strident and threatened to encompass the candidates and the training, and it seemed that there might be a permanent rupture in the British Society. In order to "pour oil on the troubled waters," as Steiner (1985) describes it, the British Society members agreed to a series of meetings to openly air their theoretical and political differences. These exchanges were named, with characteristic British reserve, the "Controversial Discussions." A long series of scientific debates took place between 1943 and 1944 in which most of the eminent psychoanalysts participated.

The results of the discussions were that each group clearly defined its theoretical positions, with each holding tenaciously to its irreconcilable views. Since the Controversial Discussions were not successful in healing the theoretical split, a gentleman's agreement or, as it has been referred to, a "ladies agreement," was drawn to ensure that both groups could coexist in the one society, teach, present their research, and supervise their students. That the British Society did not split is a testament to the determination of its members to find compromise solutions. Even Freud said that only the future would bring in a verdict on the controversial debate.

The actual compromise was worked out in the sphere of training with the formation of three groups. The middle group originally wanted to maintain its independence from the other groups and from the constraints of a fixed theoretical position without political organization. Ironically, this group constituted the majority in the British Society after the Controversial Discussions. In the 1960s it finally became an organized group in order to participate in the institutional life of the society.

The new curriculum finally drawn up in 1946, after much debate and discussion, provided for two parallel sets of lectures/seminars on technique, one with teachers from all groups, including the Kleinians, and another taught by the Anna Freud group. All other studies would be common to all students. Although there were officially only two groups, the Society was semiofficially divided into three groups. Candidates were encouraged to resist the natural tendency to identify completely with one group or another. With the passage of time, the curriculum has been modified to allow greater freedom and choice, and candidates have been supported in their efforts to obtain greater knowledge of one another's thinking. Ten years ago the term *"Contemporary"* was appended to the Freudian group to differentiate itself from the other two groups, both of which consider themselves to be Freudian. To this day the groups maintain their individuality, living in peaceful coexistence while "on some issues, dissent and conflict still rumble on," as Steiner (1985) points out. The spirit of the gentleman's agreement, however, still pervades the educational process and the Society, and as the following chapters demonstrate, the affective consequences of these historical events are still palpable.

## Reference

Steiner, R. (1985). Some thoughts about tradition and change arising from an examination of the British Psycho-Analytical Society's Controversial Discussions (1943–1944). *International Review of Psycho-Analysis* 12(1):27–71.

# II

## ANALYSTS IN SESSION: THE BRITISH PSYCHO-ANALYTICAL SOCIETY

# 3

# An "Oedipal" Session: The Contemporary Freudian Analyst

The task of finding an "oedipal" session for presentation was far from easy. Possibly this was due to my own technical approach, which although rooted in developmental thinking, gives priority to the analysis of the "here and now," with reconstruction in terms of the specific patient's development being used to provide a temporal dimension to the patient's insight. Moreover, the concept of the infantile neurosis as central to the understanding of the patient's current disturbance has fallen by the wayside. The concept of the transference neurosis is practically never used; rather, British psychoanalysts tend, from the beginning of the analysis, to think of transference manifestations in the here and now of the session.

For me the awareness of the tremendous importance of preoedipal factors also contributed to the difficulty in finding an oedipal session for this meeting. Preoedipal factors inevitably color oedipal conflicts, which we seldom see in pure culture. In my experience, truly neurotic patients are a rarity in analysis, and not all conflicts relating to the triangular situation are necessarily oedipal in quality.

The patient, Dr. A., a physician specializing in internal medicine, came to analysis three years ago at the age of 35. He was married, had two children, and had asked for help in regard to feelings of depression and isolation and a general feeling of dissatisfaction with life. Although he was performing his work well, he had been experiencing a sense of aimlessness and was having some marital difficulties that were causing him and his wife concern.

Dr. A. had settled well into five-times weekly analysis, and in the first three years considerable work had been done on his feelings of self-consciousness and anxiety about exposure and the associated fears of humiliation. All of these feelings and fears had entered and had been taken up in the transference, and Dr. A.'s symptoms had diminished considerably. There had been great improvement in his relationship to his wife, and they were now getting on well.

The session presented here occurred on a Monday. Dr. A. arrived about ten minutes before his session was due to start and was seated in the waiting room reading when I came to fetch him. He seemed somewhat startled by my entrance, gave me an embarrassed smile, and followed me up the stairs to my consulting room. He lay down on the couch as usual and, after a short silence, said, "You have a cold. You sound as if your sinuses are bunged up."

(This was in fact true. I was suffering from the after-effects of a cold and still had some catarrh.) At this point I coughed, and Dr. A. commented, "And you have a postnasal drip. You look tired and I don't want to tire you further. Perhaps I ought not to have come today."

(I did not feel that this was an intrusive comment, as I have done with some patients. Rather, I felt that what Dr. A. said was a reflection of genuine concern. However, what his remark evoked in me was a feeling that I had done something wrong, and I felt somewhat guilty at having exposed my patient to possible infection. I wondered to myself whether I should have canceled the session and thought of a conversation with my husband the previous evening in which he had urged me to take more care of myself and to think of canceling my morning patients. I had felt that I would not need to do this as the worst of my cold was over.)

Dr. A. proceeded to tell me that he had seen an attractive woman enter the house just before he had, and she had gone into the waiting room just ahead of him. He felt a little uncomfortable in her presence. My husband, with whom I share the waiting room, had come very soon to collect the woman, who Dr. A. thought might be a new patient whom he had not seen before. He commented that my husband had looked distant and rather disdainful, appearing less friendly than usual. Dr. A. wondered aloud whether my husband was annoyed that he had come early for his session. (I felt that the patient was rather hesitant and not quite comfortable as he told me this.)

After a pause Dr. A. remarked that his neck was playing him up. It felt stiff again, and he had some difficulty driving his car as he couldn't turn his neck around when reversing out of his garage. He thought he ought to visit his osteopath again for manipulation, which had been very effective on a previous occasion.

There was a further pause. Then Dr. A. said, "I had a dream last night. Stephanie (his wife) was walking along a path toward me. She was wearing a beautiful nightdress and looked very attractive. She smiled at me and I was glad to see her. But I woke up feeling quite anxious, and I couldn't understand why." He thought a while and then said, "Stephanie looked a little different from usual in the dream. She had short hair, and when I think of it, she reminded me of a photograph I have of my mother when she was young." Dr. A. then recalled an early nightmare that he had had when he was about 12, after he had gone to the circus with his parents. He dreamed he was in bed in his room when suddenly the door opened and a large tiger, just like the one that had jumped in the ring at the circus, burst into the room. Since then he had often thought of the image of this tiger, which filled him with horror. He was really very scared of it.

(As Dr. A. recounted his dream, I immediately recalled that I had been to the hairdresser the previous week and had my hair cut rather short. I now felt that Dr. A. was bringing in oedipal material, which had not been much in evidence in the analysis before. He was clearly somewhat anxious and less relaxed than usual, and I had the feeling that behind this emotion was some excitement. I wondered whether the tiger represented some sadistic and frightening aspect of his self. I decided to wait before offering an interpretation, as I was not sure what had prompted all this material and why it was coming to the surface during this particular session.)

Dr. A. then said, rather hesitatingly, that he and Stephanie had wanted to make love the previous night. He had felt like doing this and was aroused, but when it came to the point he could not sustain his erection. This had happened only once or twice before. Stephanie was sympathetic and had gone down on him, taking his penis into her mouth and sucking him. He did not get a full erection, but ejaculated suddenly into her mouth. He said that he was sure that Stephanie would be angry, but she laughed and had simply said, "It had a funny taste." He went on to say, "This had never happened to me before. Immediately afterward I thought of having to tell you about it today. I kept asking Stephanie if she was all right, but she did not seem to mind at all."

(I now felt convinced that what I had sensed in the session was his excitement linked to sexual fantasies in the transference. It seemed clear to me that there was a connection between what he said about ejaculating into Stephanie's mouth and his comment about his stiff neck and my bunged-up sinuses and postnasal drip. However, I decided to wait before interpreting his unconscious sexual wishes toward me fully to be sure I could do so in an emotionally convincing manner, particularly as Dr. A. had a tendency at times to use intellectualization as a defense. Accordingly, I limited myself to saying, "When I think of your dream, and what happened with Stephanie last night, I cannot help but feel that in your mind Stephanie, your mother, and I were all mixed up.")

Dr. A. was silent for some minutes and said, "I do seem to have women on my mind. I wasn't very comfortable with that woman in the waiting room. I was trying not to pay attention to her, but she was very attractive. I was turning over the pages of a magazine and had just turned to an article about beauty contests when your husband came in. I don't think he saw what I was looking at, but I was terribly embarrassed, and I wondered what he thought. At that moment I felt sure he disapproved of me."

After a further silence Dr. A. said, "I still feel ashamed so easily. I remember when I was a boy I stayed home from school one day because I had a cold. My mother let me lie on my parents' bed, and I was supposed to be doing some reading for school. But I didn't really feel like doing that, and I started to look at a magazine I found in the room. It had a separate brochure in it with advertisements for brassieres, and I remember that I was quite excited. I got a shock when my father walked into the room—he had come home from work early, and I felt very embarrassed in case he had seen what I was reading. Actually, I had an erection at the time. But he seemed not to have noticed it and was very solicitous. He had brought me some comics.

"Actually, Dad was a nice man, although at times he could be very strict. Mother was more indulgent, but I think she was really afraid of Dad. When I was naughty she did not want to punish me, but Dad would insist that she did. I was spoiled by her, really." The patient now fell silent.

At this point I recalled that at the end of Friday's session I had felt very warm toward Dr. A. and pleased with the progress of his analysis. I had looked forward to his next hour.

This seemed to me to be a countertransference clue to the oedipal theme that was developing in Dr. A.'s material, and I felt it appropriate to say, "On Friday you told me you were very pleased with the way our work was going. You told me of the promotion you had been offered and that you felt how much you had changed because of our analytic work. I think that these feelings made you rather scared and that you became afraid that my husband would resent the fact that you and I were getting on so well."

Dr. A. responded by saying, "I don't know about your husband, but over the weekend I was concerned about Dr. X. (a colleague of his) because I was promoted over his head. He was angry, I know, and snubbed me in the dining room on Friday. I want to make my peace with him, although I would be far happier if he left the hospital. He is the sort of person who bears a grudge, and I don't trust him. I think I must have been feeling rather guilty about the promotion because on Saturday morning I managed to bash in the wing of my car when I drove out of the driveway—I've driven out of the drive thousands of times before, without any accident." (Dr. A. had insight into the fact that when he felt guilty he tended to have minor accidents—mislaying keys, forgetting appointments, and the like.)

I commented, "Perhaps there is a part of you that would like to have my husband out of the way so that you can have me all to yourself. But I think that this makes you uneasy, and so you feel the need to make your peace with him too."

Dr. A. laughed and said, "Yes, I'd like to. I'd hate to feel that I had a hostile husband just around the corner." He was silent for a minute and then said, "I have to visit my nephew Jack—he's had his operation and is doing well. It's funny that I also had a hernia when I was 5—it must run in the family. The surgeon was a friend of my father, but I remember that I was scared of the operation, although my mother was with me all the time. I remember looking at the scar when they changed the dressing. It seemed an enormous wound. Afterward I kept trying to look at it. In fact you can hardly see it now."

I remarked, "You must have been terribly frightened then, and I think that when you say you looked at the scar you must also have been checking up on your 'willy' [the patient's word for his penis] to see if it was still there. I think thoughts about Jack's operation and your own came to your mind just now because of a fear that my husband would revenge himself for your excitement about his female patient and about me, that he would punish and emasculate you for daring to want him out of the way. But I think that all of this has been triggered by your promotion—you've been more successful than your father was, and we know that you have been very guilty about that. We also know that you are aware of the fact that you can allow yourself to do better because of our work here, but it scares you—it is as if you take my husband's women away from him—his patient and me—and in the past your father's woman, your mother. So you expect punishment."

This was the end of the session.

# 4

## A Session Illustrating Severe Oedipal Pathology and Difficulties with Termination: The Independent Analyst

It is common practice for writers in psychoanalysis, especially those writing about clinical issues and problems of technique, to justify their case presentation by drawing attention to how little has previously been written about the topic. I do so myself as well. Since Freud's paper, "Psychoanalysis Terminable and Interminable" (1937), there have been few papers on the subject and very few on the techniques for bringing about the ending of analysis. Freud's more general guides, such as "transforming what is unconscious to what is conscious" or "where id was there shall ego be," or that an ending is possible when self-analysis replaces psychoanalysis, as useful as they are, help little in managing the ending of a present-day analysis.

Harold Blum (1989) wryly comments that self-analysis does not deal with termination. Freud did not take leave of himself. Blum adds that this may be the reason Freud—the self analyst—even when he discussed object loss in *Mourning and Melancholia*—did not refer to the loss of the analyst. Freud wrote (1937), "Whatever one's theoretical attitude to the question may be, the termination of an analysis is, I think, a practical matter" (p. 249). And in a letter to Fliess he wrote of a long analysis he was conducting: "I would have continued the treatment, but I had the feeling that such prolongation is a compromise between illness and health that patients themselves desire, and the physician therefore must not accede to it." (Masson 1985, p. 409)

In the early years, Freud often set time limits for the ending of analysis, most famously perhaps in the case of the Wolf Man, to whom he gave a final six months. Freud writes, "Under the inexorable pressure of a fixed limit his resistance gave way and the analysis produced all the material which made it possible to clear up his inhibitions and remove his symptoms" (1918, p. 11). Blum's (1989) criticism of analysts who set fixed termination dates in an attempt to uncover hidden pathology is "Shit or get off the pot" or "Shape up or ship out" (p. 281). In "Psychoanalysis Terminable and Interminable" Freud also writes that fixing time limits is akin to blackmail that produced some material and repressed other. Ferenczi, writing in 1927 on the problem of termination of analysis, says, "Analysis is not terminated by the analyst or the patient. It dies of exhaustion" (p. 85).

Leo Rangell (1966), in "An Overview of the Ending of an Analysis," reminds us that disappointment and disillusionment are usually felt in the posttermination phase. "There are inherent real limitations of the patient, analyst, and the analytic process" (cited in Blum 1989, p. 287). Some hopes and dreams can never be fulfilled. Termination leads to a new confrontation with magical expectations and infantile omnipotence, and one should not conclude that terminal disturbance always means the need for more analysis. The anticipated loss of the analyst may induce mourning, but some patients cannot tolerate the anticipated separation. For them the analysis is not over until it is over.

From whom does the patient terminate, the real person-analyst or the tranference object? Rangell writes, "The analyst is primarily mourned as transference object. Loss of the analysing object of the analysis, is also mourned but not in the depth and poignancy of the transference object loss. We never reach the Promised Land." (Blum 1989, pp. 291, 293).

Mrs T. was 40ish, a teacher who had had five years' therapy earlier following a severe postdivorce depression. Sensitive, articulate, and masochistic, she had not been allowed to work by her husband, who was very successful. She dutifully looked after the children, who were now grown up and were high achievers. The father had left her for other relationships several years earlier, but he maintained contact.

Overall, Mrs T. was very sad, unable to cope with losses, and in a state of chronic mourning. She was often briefly hypomanic, with moments of elation and overactivity. She also had psychosomatic symptoms often seen in cyclothymic patients, and keeping her weight down was a problem.

Her middle-class and educated father became ill before she was born, and although he lived until she became an adult, he was severely restricted as a father, husband, and worker. The mother became the breadwinner, and the home was deeply sad, dominated by the father's illness and with no other children and few visitors. She was often sent to other relatives for both short and long periods so that the mother could care for the father, whose illness, she was told, would get worse if she was "naughty" or noisy. Playful interaction with Father was not available because of his fragility and his very limited capacity to communicate.

### Main Features in the Analysis

Mrs T., despite her sophistication and psychological minded-ness, was from the start relentlessly in search of the real person behind my professional mask. She resented interpretations that she saw as proof of my uncaringness. She began almost every session by expressing her wish not to come, but she never asked questions about me because she could not bear rejection. She never gave up the hope of a warm, caring relationship with a man in a position of authority, and she was excited and triumphant if she could discern any trace of "weakness" in me, such as a lapse of memory or being slightly late. Weaknesses meant that I was human; the perfect analytic stance reminded her of her masklike unresponsive father. The wish to end the analysis led partly from these considerations. Perhaps after it was all over we could relate in a different way (although she knew too that we could not, and at bottom, she did not wish it either). She set several termination dates, giving a few months' notice; each time even the most tentative consensus precipitated a deepening depression, silences, and weight gain. She was convinced I could not wait to see her go, but her greatest fear was that if she did not take control of the ending she would come forever, in a helpless state, and that I would be helpless too and would be unable to do anything about it. After this pattern was repeated several times over several years, I told her about a month before the most "real" last date that she should remain in therapy for another full year. This was based on advice given by Michael Balint many years ago about a patient with similar termination pathology. She protested vehemently; it was cruel. Prisoners receive a remission of sentence, not another year. But despite her angry rejection of my proposal, she accepted it the next day, and there followed considerable relief and the most productive year of the entire analysis. Most of all it undercut her most tenaciously held beliefs from the start—that I never really wanted her as a patient and that I secretly wished to replace her with a more worthwhile patient.

Throughout the analysis she exhibited intense competitiveness with me, anticipating my interpretations (especially of dreams) and leaping in when she discerned the direction of my thinking. Her actions were impelled by a conscious wish that I recognize how bright she was, an experience she never had with her parents, who took no interest in her school progress. She had a particular longing to bring pleasure and pride to her father, in part because the coincidence of his illness and her birth left her feeling that she had been responsible for his severely disabled state.

## The Session

This was a Thursday session, a few months before the end. The letters T.I. stand for Therapeutic Intervention.

*Mrs. T.:* "I did something quite shameful today. It gave me an excited voyeuristic feeling. I saw a mother at my school. She had sexually abused her 5-year-old child. When she was a teenager she was abused sexually, and she was sent to the Tavistock, to see a man with red hair and glasses. She said he wasn't much good. I at once felt excited, and I later rang the Tavistock to ask who saw the child (it was you) and if the patient had been seen for consultation or treatment. I hoped it was treatment, because I would feel more triumphant if you were a useless therapist, but you had only seen the patient once. Still, I felt superior, especially as you were considered an expert in child sexual abuse cases. The patient also said you were tubby. You are not that now, but I felt indignant that you made interpretations about the self-destructiveness of my being overweight when you were once tubby yourself. I was going to ask the Tavistock for a copy of your report, but I didn't think they would give it and anyway it seemed too intrusive. What made it worse was that a month ago I saw a family with a history of incest who saw you five or six years ago at the Tavistock, and they said you had been very helpful. I did not know if it was a consultation or therapy because I did not want to be made envious, and I did not tell you what the patient said because I did not want to make you feel proud. I am much more interested in hearing bad than good things about you. It shows what a bitch I am beneath my genteel facade."

*T.I.:* "You have a need for idols, but you find it exciting when they fall, as Father did."

*Mrs. T.:* "I never told you, but from the age of 3 until I was evacuated at 4½ (referring to the evacuation of London during World War II) I was a severe head-banger."

*T.I.:* "Perhaps in identification with Father's 'turns.' And if I 'fall' or fail by being a useless consultant, I seem to be the father, always liable to fall."

*Mrs. T.:* "When I began analysis I thought you might be weak. I even thought in my arrogance that I would teach you. But you were stronger than I thought, wouldn't stand any nonsense, and you always seemed to see through my tricks. I have never felt even a ripple of emotion from you, apart from a certain slight irritation in your voice occasionally, so I never worry about upsetting you. I often upset my previous therapist, and I had her in tears once. On another occasion she told me all about *her* mother's death. Although I was gratified at the time, I felt angry afterward, especially as she was charging me for listening to her problems."

*T.I.:* "So you felt you could tell me about my useless consultation without fearing I would be in tears."

*Mrs. T.:* "Well, we all do bad consultations sometimes."

*T.I.*: "You are reassuring me now, but also managing to say, 'We are all the same.'"

*Mrs. T.*: "Yes, I am as good as you. I may be a child, but I'm as good as a parent."

*T.I.*: "I think your search for weakness in men (husband, father, me) is not only a wish to triumph but also to find a weak father to at last replace Mother and you can look after the weak father."

*Mrs. T.*: "Mother told me every night to say a prayer for Father, because he might die."

*T.I.*: "You probably also believed it was you, by your birth or your badness, who caused his illness."

*Mrs. T.*: "Yes, but whatever about that fantasy, it was also true that I caused it. Without me it would not have happened."

*T.I.*: "Today, you show how much you need to make me the father who is knocked down (the bad consultation), but then also, quickly revived (by reporting the good consultation)."

*Mrs. T.*: "There was a song, 'You pick me up and then you let me down.' I let you down, to pick you up. My sad feelings are less. I have not been thinking of the ending in funeral terms. It is more like graduation day. Yesterday I went to the funeral of a colleague's husband. It was a humanist service—readings from Shakespeare and Donne. I'd like that kind of funeral for me. One line I recall was 'Don't hope to arise from the dead.' After 16 years—almost half with you, I must be a slow learner. I do not believe in an afterlife, but I now believe in a psychoanalytic afterlife. I had been building a paranoid structure around myself, like scaffolding, to shore up a shaky edifice inside. I wanted to spend the rest of my life licking my wounds, abandoned by everyone. Although I set the pace for the several premature terminations, they could easily have been viewed later as being abandonment by you, just like all the others. The extra year, and especially its timing, stripped away the scaffolding and negated my favorite stance, that I was unloved and unlovable. I think it gave me hope."

*Silence.* "I'm now thinking of graduation day. I want to say to you, 'Didn't we do well?' But I also feel nothing has changed. I'm still the same person I always was."

T.I.: "Perhaps you are saying, 'Haven't we done well to avoid change.'"

*Mrs. T.:* "That seems silly and wrong, because much *has* changed. But I'm glad I am still the same person. One symptom that I've had all my adult life is waking up, as from a nightmare, with the thought, 'I haven't done it,' 'I've forgotten something,' 'It's too late now.' I can't tell you how real that was—we've often spoken about it. In the past six months it has greatly faded, and it is now quite benign—like 'Did I feed the cat last night' or 'Did I leave out a note for extra milk?' But before my failure was unspecified and it was like a nameless dread, accompanied by massive guilt. Now I enjoy waking up." (In this last year she had managed at last to reduce her weight by two stone from 15 to 13 stone. She had also taken up swimming, which she had last done sixteen years earlier on the last family holiday before her marriage broke up.)

*Silence.* "In a way I feel strange, rather cut off, sad and happy. I've never enjoyed swimming so much as in the last month. I love the freedom to move around. I'm glad I had some lessons from the instructor."

*T.I.*: "I'm the instructor who helped you to swim."

*Mrs. T.*: "I don't think you ever instructed me, or showed me how to do anything. I feel you are the water."

## My Thoughts During the Session

The opening material, of triumphing over me and then restoring me, was extremely familiar. She was drawn to very potent men, especially intellectually, but she was overjoyed to discover their weaknesses, especially sexually: "Boys will be boys." She was ignored by her mother, who never forgave her, and she loved her father from afar. She repeated this in the transference, seeing me as both strong and weak. She identified with a very morose father, lacking spontaneity, and she was herself internally dead, always completely anorgasmic, and terrified that sexual excitement stood for or could provoke a seizure. She had a specific fear of urinary incontinence in intercourse. She knew quite early that this usually happened to Father.

She desperately wanted a "well" father; while she indulged in manic reparation in relation to the rejecting mother, her transference wish was to make me well. Yet she also knew how intensely rivalrous she was with me. She knew that Father's needs deprived her of a mother, and Mother's slavish nursing devotedness deprived her of a father. She felt she could deal with this conflict either by running away prematurely or staying forever. I decided I had to take control and to give her enough time.

The most significant statement she ever made was when, in this session, she said that after sixteen years she accepted that her marriage was at an end. There were plenty of indications of moves to an ending, but it would hardly be possible to convey the intensity of her longing to be back in the marriage, for all its limitations and cruelties. She had to reach a point of letting go of the marriage before she could let go of me.

But to the end, she was able to challenge and disagree. On the very last session she told me that on the morning she was going into the nursing home to have her last child, her husband told her he was leaving her and that he would be gone when she returned from the nursing home. On the fourth day the pediatrician told her the baby had an infection. "Poor little thing," she said. "Perhaps he knows he won't have a Daddy." I interpreted that she was telling me that she was the Poor Little Thing who did not have a Daddy and the analysis was also a Poor Little Thing who is no longer going to have me as a Daddy. In response she said, "But the analysis is not a Poor Little Thing—it's a bouncing baby."

Ernst Ticho (1972) divides termination into two phases: (1) agreement that the analysis should terminate and (2) the setting of the date proper. During these phases, he advises *against* any change of technique such as abandoning the couch or reducing the frequency of sessions. He adds that, as the transference neurosis is resolved, the analyst emerges as a more real person, and it is unwise for the analyst to do anything to reinforce this. The first move to terminate should come from the patient, but the decision to terminate should be a joint one. The analyst ought not reassure the patient that he will be available for consultation later, as this conveys doubts about the patient's capacity to cope.

John Klauber, in his 1977 paper "Analysis that Cannot Be Terminated," makes the point that difficulty in terminating is usually associated with deep early maternal deprivation. Such patients are unable to come to terms with object loss, but they mobilize in their analysts a powerful and often unconscious wish to keep them. This may lead to analytic paralysis and interminable analysis. Klauber maintains that the patient should always initiate a proposal to terminate. But what if the patient avoids every means and has no intention ever to terminate? One of my patients, who stayed in therapy for fifteen years, would become totally silent in response to any mention of termination by me and eventually angrily shouted, "I came to you for analysis, not to discuss the ending of the analysis. Why do you not get on with the analysis? The analysis will end when it ends." Then there are those, like Mrs. T., who talk incessantly about ending the analysis as a longed-for goal but who show by their reaction to any serious consideration of ending that they are terrified of any *actual* ending.

## Some Comments on the Session Material and Alternative Interpretations Not Given

The opening material in the session is very rich, with elements of excitement about her discovery of my past secret professional life, in which I am bad (impotent) but also good (potent). She acknowledges her jealousy and her wish to be destructively attacking. I present this session because it represents a feature of a great many sessions in which I am supposed to be good but turn out to be bad. I had interpreted all this material on countless occasions very negatively, as illustrative of her sadism, her longing for a powerful penis that she can demolish with triumph and manic elation. This time I focused on the reparative wish to find Father wanting so that she can then take over Mother's function to care for and rehabilitate him. I did this because we were so near the end and because I had previously noted that too much emphasis on her destructiveness led to a worsening of her clinical depression.

# References

Blum, H. P. (1989). The concept of termination and the evolution of psychoanalytic thought. *Journal of the American Psychoanalytic Association* 37(2):275–295.

Ferenczi, S. (1927). The problem of the termination of the analysis. In *Final Contributions to the Problems and Methods of Psycho-Analysis*, pp. 77–86. New York: Brunner/Mazel, 1980.

Freud, S. (1917a). Mourning and melancholia. *Standard Edition* 14.

—— (1917b). Introductory lectures on psycho-analysis. *Standard Edition* 16.

—— (1918). From the history of an infantile neurosis. *Standard Edition* 17.

—— (1933). New introductory lectures on psycho-analysis. *Standard Edition* 22.

Klauber, J. (1977). Analyses that cannot be terminated. *International Journal of Psycho-Analysis* 58:473–477.

Masson, J., ed. (1985). *The Complete Letters of Sigmund Freud to Wilhelm Fliess—1887–1904*. Cambridge, MA: Harvard University Press.

Rangell, L. (1966). An overview of the ending of an analysis. In *Psychoanalysis in America*, ed. R. E. Litman, pp. 141–173. New York: International Universities Press.

Ticho, E. E. (1972). Termination of psychoanalysis: treatment goals, life goals. *Psychoanalytic Quarterly* 41:315–333.

# 5

# A Session with Mrs. D.:
# The Modern Kleinian Analyst

The patient is a professional woman in her mid-thirties who has been in analysis with me for three years. She is married and has two small children; the marriage seems to be a good one. She comes from a large Scottish family and is the eldest of five children. She came to analysis complaining of mild but chronic depression, a sense of purposelessness, and various vague physical complaints that seemed to be psychosomatic. Recently the patient had been complaining about a pain in her arm and shoulder; sometimes this was severe enough to keep her from going to her job.

The analysis has been occasionally quite stormy; the patient can be irritable, argumentative, and critical, but she also values her analysis and the help she feels it has given her.

The session presented here took place on the Friday of the first week after my summer break. The patient couldn't get to the first session of the week because of problems with her child care arrangements; she had phoned the night before, very upset. She arrived late and distressed to the second session, complaining about the traffic (she lives about 1½ hours outside London). In the following sessions that week she spoke about feeling miserable over the long summer break, but, she kept insisting, with no good reason. She said she was feeling a mess. She had imagined me over the summer—what was I doing? The sessions felt disconnected and frustrating, and there was a lack of real contact between us.

The consulting room had been redecorated over the summer; there is new striped wallpaper. The patient hasn't mentioned it.

I kept her waiting three minutes. She lay down and spoke about the traffic: it was absolutely horrible today! She doesn't understand it; whichever way she tries to get here there is traffic, and it's blocked up and difficult. She tried to take a new route—but once she got round the corner it was completely blocked up.

(I knew she was talking about a real, external event, but I felt sure she also was speaking about her response to being kept waiting.)

I said that I thought my keeping her waiting this morning was horrible for her, that she feels that there has been some kind of traffic in this room that has blocked her access to me and made her feel how really difficult she feels it is to actually get back to me.[1]

She was silent for a moment. Then, in an irritated voice, she said that in the waiting room she *had* been panicky. She'd wondered: Did she have the wrong time or was I not going to be here? She felt worried and panicky. She feels in a mess—she's so confused—and has felt in a mess all week. She then suddenly added in a different voice, "But it's silly, of course

---

1. After reading the commentaries, I thought it important to emphasize that I do not often interpret this early in the session. However, I was aware that this was a Friday, that the patient had been frustrated and not contactable all week, and I thought it was important to try to make immediate contact with her if I could. I was prepared to follow my hunch because I know from past experience how jittery and distressed this patient becomes when I am late and because the sessions from earlier in the week were permeated by a sense of her frustration about not being able to get back to me.

I'm not really in a mess. It's just that I feel ashamed of feeling bad—but how ridiculous, what nonsense, nothing is actually wrong, it's ridiculous to feel this way."

(This last comment *was* in a different voice: cold, critical, superior, and off-putting. She didn't sound like herself, and I felt suddenly distanced from her and put down.)

I said I thought she had been trying to tell me how she feels, but that something then had come along inside her and interfered.

She was silent for a moment and then began rubbing her arm, saying how painful her arm and shoulder have been and that the pain is certainly one of the things making her feel bad and confused—if she could choose what to get rid of, she would get rid of the pain in her arm!

(My immediate feeling was of inadequacy—she was really hurt by the pain in her arm that I was unable to do anything to cure. I felt uncomfortably useless. I thought a little more, and began to feel that this feeling of being useless had, a moment before, been hers when she was being berated by herself in such a strict voice. I then began to think that there is something she wants fervently to get rid of, and it seemed to be experienced as the pain in her arm.)

She looked at the new wallpaper in the room and rubbed her finger on the stripe, referring to the fact that the room had been redecorated in her absence over the summer. (This was the first reference made to the redecoration.) She said it reminded her of the wallpaper in "Woodside House," a house her family had lived in when she was small, before the age of 8. She had shared a bedroom with her brother for awhile, and it had paper very much like this, with stripes. She shared the room while the nursery was being redecorated, she thinks. (I know that by this time in her life there were three children in the family and the fourth was on the way. As mentioned above, the patient is the oldest of five children.) She has funny memories of that bedroom. She used to spoil the wallpaper by licking her finger and rubbing the spit on the wall—it made terrible marks because the paper was striped, she guesses, and not patterned. She paused. She also remembered that she spilled cod-liver oil in her bed, all over the sheets. Her mother was extremely cross and shouted at her. However, a few years ago she mentioned this memory to her mother, and her mother said that was nonsense, that she, Mother, would never have been cross about such a thing.

This bedroom, the patient went on, was at the other end of the corridor from her parents' bedroom; it was at the corner end of the house and jutted out and over into another house's garden, so that in fact it was as if it was a part of the other house. The house next door was owned by the Irwins. When she was in the bedroom, she felt as if she was in the other people's house.

(At this point I was thinking that she was telling me about memories into which she had been plunged by the situation between us—that she was talking about where she is in her mind when she feels I am at the far end of a long corridor from her—because of the holidays, because of keeping her waiting. I felt aware that in the consulting room there was a little girl and somewhere in her mind there is a mother and father together, and that she is doing something messing up with her finger, and that this leads to a thought about being inside the "other people's house." I felt these were important memories stimulated by the events within the analysis.)

She then said that she remembers masturbating in bed in this room, under the covers. She notes that she has told me about this before: she worked herself up "into a lather." Her father came in, she had expected him to be excited by her excited sweatiness, but instead he was angry and disgusted with her.

(I had been thinking that she was talking about masturbation before she had mentioned it—partly of course because she had told me about it before. I now had to think about what I thought was going on in the session. I considered whether I thought there was a kind of masturbation going on right then and there, in which I was expected to find her memories "exciting." I thought this might be true, but I did not think it was of primary importance. What I did think was important was her description of what she does when she feels far away from her parents. I thought that she was vividly describing a painful situation into which she had been thrown by my lateness coming on top of the recent summer holiday.)

I said that when I was late it made her feel that something or someone was keeping me away from her—was interfering with her getting to me. I thought *that* was what was hurting her and that she experienced it not so much in her feelings as in her arm. And I thought that when she came into the room and became aware of its being redecorated, it hit her with a bang—that someone else had been with me, inside of me, occupying me, and doing things with and to me while she had to wait.

She was silent for a moment and then quietly said, "Yes." (I was impressed by this affirmation because Mrs. D. does not agree openly with me very often.) I felt she was listening to me so I went on. I said that I thought that when she was in the waiting room, and then when she'd come into the room, she had felt very much the way she described feeling when she was a little girl. I think she wants to mess me up, like smearing the wallpaper and messing the bed, partly because she's angry with me, but mostly because she would much rather imagine herself as the messer-upper, the main person, than to feel as left out as she feels when she thinks someone else is here with me, "messing me up." I said I thought when she feels someone else is with me it makes her feel impossibly left out and jealous.

(When the patient had talked about messing up the

wallpaper and about soiling the bed, I had at first thought she might be talking about angry attacks, when she was little, on her parents in their bed and now on me. But as she spoke further, I began to feel that the primary anxiety was of feeling left out, with all the emotions that brings with it—loneliness, jealousy, a sense of being of no importance and forgotten about—and I thought the anger and the activity she engaged in were defensive against this anxiety.)

She said, "It's funny, you know. The room I was describing, in Woodside House. It is the room where I learned the 'facts of life.'" A little girlfriend had been playing in the room with her and had told her the facts of life, and she had become very excited. But she had completely misunderstood her friend's explanation: she thought her parents needed some kind of tube to have sexual intercourse, as if there was no penis, so she'd said to the friend, "Let's play Mummies and Daddies, I've got a tube in the cupboard we can use." And she'd gone to the cupboard to get the tube. She hadn't understood at all.

I said I think it feels terrible for her to feel like the little girl at the end of the corridor, or in the waiting room. I said I think that, when that happens, she switches things around in her mind—she imagines herself as the Daddy, the one who gets to be with the Mummy.

She said, "I've just remembered a dream . . . from last night." In her dream, she was with "that student," a male student in her course on whom she had had a crush the previous year, and they were having an affair. Although there was nothing sexual in the dream, it was established that they were having an affair and in love. And she felt tremendous happiness, just a great, great pleasure inside herself. She pointed to her breastbone—there was a light, happy feeling here. I was around somewhere in the background. She woke suddenly, feeling tremendously happy, with the feeling still there—it was the middle of the night—and she realized that she didn't have the pain in her arm and shoulder. It had gone, and she was so relieved. She lay there trying to think the dream thoughts, to get back into the dream, but she couldn't do it. She got up to go to the toilet, and when she came back to bed she realized that the pain in her arm had come back—she doesn't know why she'd had to reach for the lavatory paper, perhaps she'd pulled it or something, but in any case it was back.

Her associations to the dream were about this young man and how her original crush on him had seemed to have so much to do with the Christmas break from analysis and seemed to be carried out "under my eyes." (The young man is someone who is in a course with her and who also works at a clinic at which I work.)

I said I thought the affair with the student in her dream felt like a love affair with me, but without sexuality and without jealousy and therefore without the messing up that makes her feel so heavy and bad inside. I said that I thought in this dream, with a student connected to me, with me in the background, she has created or found the "tube" that would enable us to be sexless but perfect lovers. I spoke about her feelings as a little girl of not having a penis and therefore having to invent a "tube" that would enable her to be close to her mother in the way she wanted. I suggested that in this dream she had created a relationship to me that made her terribly happy, that was not spoiled by the presence of a father, and was therefore one in which jealousy is left out. I thought this got rid of the pain of jealousy from her mind—and therefore from her arm.

She said that yesterday she had felt terribly sad because she'd suddenly thought, "What's the use—in the end all I can be to her is her patient." Wanting to be close to me and then feeling, "Yes, but all she is is my analyst—she'll never really love me."

I said that the dream seemed to offer a cure for that sadness—no wonder she wanted so much to hold onto it in the night.

She was quiet for awhile and then spoke, in a musing kind of way, about this childhood bedroom and how it overlooked the Irwins' house and garden. She remembered playing with the Irwin girls—there were only girls in the family, all of whom were older than her, and she had often wanted to be a part of that family instead of her own. She remembers that the oldest Irwin girl used to swing her around by her arm, and once she really hurt her shoulder—she in fact pulled it out. Annie, the patient's daughter, hurt *her* shoulder over the holiday: she fell down in the caravan in which the family was staying. The patient's sister, who was also there, said that Annie is just identified with the patient—my patient said she thought that was silly.

It was the end of the session.

## Comments

My keeping the patient waiting for her session, coming as it did so soon after the long, difficult summer break and added to by the fact that the room had been redecorated in her absence, plunged this patient into an intensely painful inverted oedipal jealousy. When she had to wait for me and wonder where I was and what I was doing, she felt left out and like a little girl down at the end of a long corridor away from her parents, whom she imagines in intercourse, making babies. So far this seems to be straightforward and classically oedipal.

Yet some aspects of the patient's material seem to need further understanding: the peculiar sense of her speaking not quite like herself early in the session, the pain she reports again in her arm, and some funny, not quite dismissible feeling I have as she tells the long story about her childhood that she has somehow turned things around: when she came into the room, a situation in which there was something felt to be going on in the room in her absence comes to be about what *she* does in the bedroom, how she messes up the walls and dirties the bed. I begin to feel she has somehow shifted positions: instead of feeling herself to be the little girl pushed out by a father who is doing things to Mother, she has, by means of projective identification, become the father.

My aim in this session was to understand her anxieties and her defensive movements away from them. In this sense, underlying everything else was her profound distress at feeling abandoned and left out. During the session she demonstrated many of the ways she uses to rid herself of such disturbing feelings, including sexual excitement (the masturbation), identifying herself with the sexual father, and imagining herself and me in a blissful nonsexual union.

# III

## COMMENTARY:
## AMERICAN ANALYSTS

# 6

# Commentary by Steven Ellman

### Introduction

Psychoanalysis has entered a period similar to the era of the Tower of Babel. However, in the Old Testament God created many languages and there was confusion. In this New Testament we use the same language and there is confusion. This psychoanalytic tower can be seen as having different effects: it makes it difficult or impossible for us to communicate, or it can be seen as a precursor to developing new concepts and ways of describing clinical experiences. It seems that many promising new efforts have begun, but the tower to some extent hinders our attempts at meaningful theoretical integrations. It is hoped that we can begin to clear up terminological differences and then focus on and clarify some of our conceptual differences.

Some recent contributions have endeavored to sidestep theoretical and clinical disagreements. Wallerstein (1990) has tried to show that, although theoretical positions may vary, when one looks at behavior in the clinical situation there are areas of convergence that have previously gone undetected. Pine (1988) has offered the view that he implicitly and at times explicitly uses different models in his clinical interventions. Obviously, Pine is advocating his approach for at least some part of the analytic community. He has tried to show the usefulness of being open to different models. However, he has not as yet specified more general ideas about when and

how one should use a given theoretical position. Thus he has
not provided guidelines or rules of correspondence on how
one is to follow the illustrations he provides. Although I am
sympathetic to Wallerstein's and Pine's perspectives, we may
be glossing over theoretical differences because of the conceptual, personal, and political difficulties surrounding our
divergent positions.

Conceptually, psychoanalysis has never fully tied together theories of technique with more general theoretical
statements. It is a daunting task to attempt to detail the relationship of theory to the clinical situation. I try to show in
the present material that theoretical differences make at least
some difference in the way in which analysis is practiced.
Theoretical orientation has even affected the type of example
that was chosen for presentation by each of the three analysts. The more general question of the relationship between
theory and technique is an issue that is fortunately beyond
the realm of this chapter. Yet it is easy to underestimate the
extent to which we are influenced by theoretical assumptions,
sometimes even ones we consciously disagree with. This can
be contrasted to the role of theory twenty-five to thirty years
ago when we overestimated the extent to which theoretical
assumptions guided us in our clinical practice.

In discussing this issue on a practical level, we all know
(or at least assume) that the personal characteristics of a clinician account for most of the variation in their clinical effi-
cacy. A good clinician from any theoretical vantage point is
better than a mediocre clinician, even though the latter may
come from one's own school of thought. Politically we are
all aware that a good deal of the acrimony in psychoanalysis
is and was based on factors that reflected issues that had as
much to do with control over institutes and societies as with
the clinical and conceptual validity of a particular position.
Given these factors, it may seem somewhat tendentious or
even bizarre to maintain that theoretical differences are

important. Nevertheless, if we wish to understand the factors that govern our clinical interventions it is quite important for us to spell out our implicit and explicit theoretical suppositions.

As a last point in this brief introduction it is important to note that most clinicians have what Sandler and Sandler (1994) have called unofficial theories. These theories may be at least in part unconscious and therefore difficult or impossible to explicate fully. This would argue all the more for as full a theoretical accounting as possible. If Sandler and Sandler are correct, then it is quite useful for a clinician to begin to have a sense of the extent to which he or she is operating in an "intuitive" manner. No one expects to function on a wholly conscious level, but it seems possible to gain some sense of the degree to which we behave in ways that are unspecified by our more formal theories.

The issues raised in this introduction bear directly on how one formulates the critique of the different oedipal sessions that each author has presented. Clearly, if one sees theoretical positions as having little to do with clinical practice, then a discussion will most likely look quite different from the following one, in which it is posited that the author's theory influenced not only how the session was conducted but also the choice of session. Although the three presenters undoubtedly chose the session they presented for many reasons, embedded in their reasons is the theory they believe in and support.

In the discussion of the presentations, I first define my understanding of the oedipal stage. Once this is done I can already feel the shadow of the Tower of Babel looming behind me. I then detail why only one of the sessions seems to me primarily oedipal in nature. In this section differences in theoretical assumptions and whether (or how) they affect our clinical work are explored. This issue leads naturally to the converse question, that is, how we work clinically and whether (or more realistically "how") our differences in technique lead to different experiences in psychoanalytic treatment.

### Brief Definition of Oedipal Phenomena

It is striking to me that when I think of the conceptualization of oedipal phenomena I go first to Freud's psychosexual stages before he developed the structural model. During this era he was introducing the concept of narcissism (Freud 1910, 1911, 1913, 1914, 1915, 1917). In 1913, after he wrote "The Disposition to Obsessional Neurosis," Freud's psychosexual stages consisted of autoerotism, narcissism, object choice (anal sadism), and object love. It is during the stage of object love that we see the efflorescing of the oedipal drama. The capacity for object love implies that one could have concern for the other and to some extent give up narcissistic concerns. To be in love renders one vulnerable. Here we have one of Freud's opposites: the opposite of loving is to be loved in return. A person's sense of self is quite vulnerable at these times. His or her self-esteem is dependent on being loved in return by another who is not part of one's self, i.e., is a differentiated object. Freud is postulating that the capacity for empathy is embedded in the development of object love. This is implied in his ideas about the nature of love and the ability to appreciate and value a person who is different and separate from one's own self (representation). (I hope I am excused for this somewhat anachronistic version of Freud's views. I do believe that my statements are all implied in his writings.)

The neurotic's capacity for object love is at the least inhibited by conflict, but part of the formation of an erotic transference, as opposed to an eroticized transference, implies the capacity for object love. Anna Freud's (1936, Sandler

1983) distinction of ego-inhibitive and ego-restrictive defenses is relevant in this discussion. We assume that neurotic
patients use mostly ego-inhibitive defenses—repression, isolation, and the like. We further expect that the failure of
defense is not experienced as a collapse of the self. To be
sure, with certain hysterical and masochistic neurotic patients
it is not always easy to gauge the severity of a proclaimed
collapse. However, certain continuities in the transference
and in the person's life lend some reassurance of stability in
the treatment situation.

I have not as yet mentioned the most cited characteristic of oedipal functioning, that is, triangulation, but as stated
by Anne-Marie Sandler (1983), triangulation can occur without necessarily implying the capacity for object love. Thus
the triangulation that Abelin (1975) noted during rapprochement is one frequently cited form of nonoedipal triangulation. In a fuller way in *The Self and the Object World* (1954,
1964), Jacobson writes about the triangulation of the preoedipal rival and the various functions that the rival serves
for the anal-stage child. This child has split the mother as
a normal occurrence in this stage and is unable to maintain
a constant object representation. In her seminal writings
Jacobson presages a good deal of the contributions of Mahler
and colleagues (1975).

In summary, triangulation can be used to preserve the
self, the mother, and the preoedipal rival (whether the
father, siblings, or a fantasy figure) and to expel and incor-
porate good and bad products. Triangulation does not necessarily imply oedipal dynamics or structure. The capacity
for object love is a necessary concomitant of oedipal dynamics despite the fact that this developed faculty may be severely
hampered by intrapsychic conflict. Thus it was not by accident that Freud focused on the erotic transference; it is a
symbolic expression of the neurotic's conflicts about object
love.

Freud's views about the etiology of neurotic, narcissistic, and psychotic conditions before the advent of the structural model did not rest solely on the dynamics of the oedipal period. Rather he had a theory of fixation points that led from the stage of object love (hysteria) to object choice (obsessive-compulsive) to various points in the stage of narcissism. Melancholia, paranoia, schizophrenia, and certain types of hypochondriacal complaints all had fixation points during the stage of narcissism (Ellman 1991). The advent of the structural theory is correlated with his new preoccupation with the oedipal period as the bedrock of psychological disorders and conflicts. His involvement with oedipal formulations is interestingly mirrored by many classical analysts, who attempt to restrict the analytic situation to patients with oedipal disorders. This has led to long debates about the question of analyzability and indeed issues about whether or not an analytic process has occurred within a given patient.

Freud's influence can be seen in the omnipresence of oedipal phenomena in Kleinian theory. One could interpret, in a somewhat loose way, that Klein experienced some pressure to see the infant-child's world in oedipal terms in order to stay within the Freudian orbit. Klein considered herself to be an (or perhaps "the") inheritor of the Freudian mantle and in any case certainly saw her discoveries as a continuation as well as an expansion of the Freudian legacy. For Kleinians, the issue of defining analyzability in terms of oedipal phenomena was somewhat alleviated since oedipal themes arise throughout virtually the child's whole infantile period. This has seemingly changed, since Kleinians, or neo-Kleinians, clinically concentrate less on early radical reconstructive statements and therefore make fewer interpretations about early oedipal phenomena. The status of Kleinian or neo-Kleinian theory is less clear on the status of early oedipal phenomena. Analysts in the United States have in a rough parallel fashion moved toward developing a greater understanding of preoedipal dynamics and have also moved away from reconstructive statements. Both in Kleinian thought and in classical psychoanalysis, there were strong pressures to analyze oedipal material. This was a Freudian legacy that was continued in remarkably different ways in both psychoanalytic traditions.

## Case Material: The Freudian Analyst

The Freudian analyst presents the only session in which there is primarily oedipal material. I think that most American analysts would agree with her that "preoedipal factors inevitably color oedipal conflicts" and that "truly neurotic patients are a rarity in analysis." This has probably always been the case. It is a psychoanalytic myth that Freud saw patients who were "truly neurotic." What we can say from reviewing his case material—both published and unpublished—is that Freud enjoyed and was willing to treat patients who could maintain a positive transference. Thus, when the patient was intellectually satisfying and could maintain a positive transference, Freud saw the patient as analyzable (Ellman 1991). When the Freudian analyst writes that the concept of the transference neurosis is never or rarely used, again I would have to agree and state that in actuality Freud wrote little about the transference neurosis. It may be that contemporary writers can provide more adequate definitions. Few modern authors, with the notable exception of Bird (1972, also Reed 1990), have embraced the concept. The idea that the infantile neurosis has fallen by the wayside, however, is a bit puzzling. If I have read this analyst correctly, she is stating that the concepts of infantile and transference neurosis are practically never used by British analysts: "Rather we [British psychoanalysts] tend from the beginning of the analysis to think of transference manifestations in the here-and-now of the session."

Let me give an example of my confusion. The patient says to her, "I remember looking at the scar when they changed the dressing. It seemed an enormous wound. Afterwards I kept trying to look at it. In fact you can hardly see it now."

The analyst responds, "You must have been terribly frightened then, and I think that when you say you looked at the scar you must also have been checking up on your 'willy' [the patient's word for his penis] to see if it was still there. I think thoughts about Jack's operation and your own came to your mind just now because of a fear that my husband would revenge himself for your excitement about his female patient and about me, that he would punish and emasculate you for daring to want him out of the way. But I think that all of this has been triggered by your promotion—you've been more successful than your father was, and we know that you have been very guilty about that." The interpretation ends with a parallel being drawn between the present, the patient taking away the analyst from her husband, to the past when, the patient wished to possess "your father's woman—your mother. So you expect punishment." The session ended with this interpretation.

It is hard to understand this interpretation in terms of the here-and-now transference or even in terms of Sandler and Sandler's (1983, 1984, 1994) theoretical ideas about the present unconscious. The interpretation offered at the end of the session is a clear example of reconstruction based on certain theoretical ideas about the early or infantile form of the patient's neurosis. There is a clear reference and assumption about the patient's castration anxiety. When the Freudian analyst talks about the patient at age 5 wondering if his willy was still there, she is making a reconstructive comment. Given Freud's influence, this type of comment is so natural that perhaps few analysts would doubt that the patient was anxious about the loss of his penis as opposed to his being worried about his scar. There are certainly equal references

to the patient's present life and his transference to the analyst, and to her husband, but reconstruction is freely mixed
with transference interpretations. This is again clearly seen
when the analyst comments on Dr. A.'s desire to possess his
mother.

There are several questions about this session that
I cannot really comment on since I do not know the case.
The analyst has written that during this session Dr. A. was
talking about oedipal material "which had not been in the
analysis before." If this is the case then why has she interpreted it so fully in this session, particularly if her criteria
for interpretation are based primarily on the here-and-now
transference.

To briefly review the case, the night before the session
the patient had a dream where the analyst seemed to be represented in a sexually alluring manner. Dr. A. had a sexual
experience with his wife in which he was unable to maintain
an erection. His wife was good natured about it "and did not
seem to mind at all" when instead of having intercourse
he prematurely ejaculated in her mouth. He immediately
thought of the analyst and then remembered an embarrass-
ing time when his mother let him lie on his parents' bed. He
remembers that his mother "did not want to punish me. . . .
I was spoiled by her, really." (His father was the punitive one.)
Is the analyst symbolically spoiling the patient by coming to
the session despite the fact that she is sick? (We must remember that she was feeling very warmly toward the patient on
Friday.) Is the patient subtly moving the analyst to protect
him, the way he wished his mother would protect him as a
child? More to the point and less speculatively, is his inabil-
ity to have sex with his wife related to his transference with
the analyst in the sense that he is trying to show her that he
is not an adult sexually? Perhaps he would rather stay the
analyst's favorite child? This seems the most direct expression of the transference, but of course it is impossible to

comment with any sense of conviction without knowing the case material more fully.

Obviously I am questioning the analyst's assertion that she focuses on the here-and-now transference and does not highlight infantile conflicts. What we see in this session is the interplay between patient and analyst that is typical in helpful analyses. The Freudian analyst understands the transference–countertransference sequences, and at some point in the treatment this material will be or perhaps already has been interpreted. What is perhaps most relevant here in this session is that when the patient had his operation, his mother "was with him all the time." The Freudian analyst is with the patient, and when the appropriate time comes she will separate from him more fully in the analysis and allow him to experience his oedipal conflicts more fully in the transference. The Freudian analyst has a clear conception of the patient's transference and the conditions of the patient's infantile neurosis; she has used these theoretical concepts to interpret both the transference and the "memories" that are relevant to the transference.

## Case Material: The Kleinian Analyst

The Kleinian analyst's session deals with a type of patient we are perhaps most familiar with in our analytic consulting rooms. The session occurred after the summer break, on the last day of the first week of sessions. The patient is having a difficult time after the break, but she relates that it is "for no good reason." The patient misses the first session and comes late to the second session. In the reported session, the analyst is three minutes late.

The patient comes in and talks about the terrible traffic. "It's blocked up, difficult." She tried to take a new route, but once she got round the corner it was completely blocked up.

The analyst comments, "I knew she was talking about a real, external event, but I felt sure she was also speaking about her responses to being kept waiting. I said I thought my keeping her waiting this morning was horrible for her, that she feels that there has been some kind of traffic in this room that has blocked her access to me and made her feel how really difficult it is to actually get back to me.

"She was silent for a moment. Then, in an irritated voice she said that in the waiting room she *had* been panicky. She'd wondered, did she have the wrong time? Or was I [the analyst] not going to be here? She felt worried and panicky. She feels in a mess—she's so confused and she has felt in a mess all week. She then suddenly added in a different voice, 'But it's silly; of course I'm not really in a mess. It's just that I feel ashamed of feeling bad—but how ridiculous, what nonsense, nothing is actually wrong. It's ridiculous to feel this way.'

"This last comment *was* in a different voice: cold, critical, superior, and off-putting. She didn't sound like herself, and I felt suddenly distanced from her and put down. I said I thought she had been trying to tell me how she feels, but that something then had come along inside her and interfered.

"She was silent for a moment and then began rubbing her arm, saying how painful her arm and shoulder have been, and that that is certainly one of the things making her feel bad and confused—if she could choose what to get rid of, she would get rid of the pain in her arm!

"My immediate feeling was of inadequacy—she was really hurt by the pain in her arm that I was unable to do anything to cure. I felt uncomfortably useless. I thought a little more, and began to feel that this feeling of being useless had, a moment before, been hers when she had berated herself in such a strict voice. I then began to think that there is something she wants fervently to get rid of, and it seemed to be experienced as the pain in her arm."

The analyst is not simply talking here about the patient waiting for three minutes, but is referring to the patient's difficulty in waiting for her over the summer break. The possible dilemma here is that, by providing a reading of the patient's feelings and thoughts before having heard the patient's response to her coming late, the analyst put the patient in a passive position. Although she has clearly made a sensitive reading of the patient's state, she may not have allowed the patient to establish—or, more accurately, re-establish—her contact with the analyst.

The patient begins to develop somatic symptoms and has a sensation that she can indisputably claim is her own experience—a pain in her arm. However, at this point the analyst feels useless and remains silent. The patient then begins to talk about the redecoration of the analyst's office.

The matter of differences in technique concerns the analyst's early interpretative efforts in this session. Based on her knowledge of the patient, the analyst determined that she knew what was happening in the patient's world. Clearly, it is difficult to sort out the complex interaction between patient and analyst because of the counterpoint between the analyst's perspective and the patient's world.

If we take the patient's perspective, it is possible to accept that on coming back from vacation she is not ready to hear the analyst's communications. Narcissistically vulnerable patients often take time to regain what I have called analytic trust (Ellman 1991), and several authors have pointed out that such patients have difficulty dealing with transitions (Bach 1985). Here, the patient seemed to have a good deal of difficulty in returning to treatment, and perhaps she felt as useless as the analyst did in the interaction recounted. The interpretation did not seem to start from an element of the patient's acknowledged experience, nor did the analyst's behavior seem to be acknowledged in this interaction. The patient may have felt it necessary to respond more on the analyst's level or risk being left out of the interaction. At first she could converse only through somatic or body language. In this interchange the theory that produced projective identification may have allowed the analyst to interpret before the patient's associations were accepted.

The patient then remembers, after noting the office redecoration, that she had made marks on the wall of her bedroom and spilled cod-liver oil on her bed. She notes that her mother shouted at her, but also says that the mother recently denied that. Is the patient remembering her mother's denial as a way of mentioning her experience of the analyst not commenting on her coming late to a session?

In another experience the patient has a memory. The bedroom was on the other end of the corridor. She remembers masturbating in bed. Her father wasn't excited by her, but rather disgusted by her. The interpretation then was that "When I was late today it made you feel something—someone was keeping me away from you—was interfering with you getting to me." I thought *that* was what was hurting her and that she experienced it in her arm.

The patient says only "yes." The analyst goes on to describe how the patient wants to mess her up rather than feel left out. Is the patient's brother a younger brother? Does the father get excited when the boy plays ball and sweats just as he gets excited when the mother sweats? She feels that "someone else is here with me, 'messing me up.'" This makes her feel impossibly left out and jealous.

In all the patient's associations there does not seem to be the jealousy the analyst talks about, but rather the wish to mess up and to be seen and felt by her parents (mother-joint parent, and so on). The excitation from the dream about the student seems like a type of hypomanic excitement, a happiness about finding the lost object that allowed her to leave all her pain and sorrow behind. The lack of sexual content in the dream, symbolized for her a state in which there would

be none of those troubling bodily feelings. These are the feeling states that disrupt her and stop her from being close to
her analyst. Then her body betrayed her (she had to go to
the bathroom), and this reminded her of her somatic (sexual)
existence and the pain came back (symbolizing her conflicts
surrounding her sexual self).

It is interesting that at the end of the session, the analyst states that the "affair with the student in her dream felt
like a love affair with me, but without sexuality and without
jealousy and therefore without the messing up." Then the
patient invented a penis to be closer to the mother. Here our
views converge about the content of the session. The patient
talks about her longing for the analyst and says that in her
view the analyst will never really love her. The patient is identified as the daughter and wants to return (or have) a blissful relationship with her mother with no one else around to
disturb her. She wants her mother (the analyst) to be there
as a continuous presence.

Is this an oedipal dynamic? I do not see this patient
functioning at the level of object love. I was impressed by
the analyst's comments that, "underlying everything else was
her [the patient's] profound distress at feeling abandoned
and left out. During the course of the session she demonstrated many of the ways she has to be rid of such disturbing
feelings." This is what I mean by the patient's body betray-
ing her: she wants to be rid of her tendencies to mess up—be
dirty, do dirty things, and so forth. She would like to give up
these pleasures for the love of her mother. She is at the point
of making an object choice[1], but she has little understand-

---

1. By object choice I am referring to the time in the child's life where
he gives up a sexual pleasure for the object in his life. Freud dated
this time in the anal stage. Others might say that this occurs during
rapproachment. In any case it is not a point of full object love but
a step toward the development of object love.

ing of her mother's (the analyst's) position. She despairs
about being able to obtain the analyst's love because she
doesn't know how to get rid of her bodily concerns. She does
not seem concerned with or conflicted about object love, nor
does her concern with her primary object seem involved with
jealousy (envy is still primary). Rather she is trying to figure
out how the preoedipal rival is allowed in the bedroom. It is
all still a mystery to her.

These various formulations are merely speculations and
my ideas may not adequately relate to the central themes in
this woman's life. This analyst knows the patient in a way that
I could never know her. Yet the form of the session is provided by a theory-driven technique that I believe reduces the
analytic space available to the patient in two instances: first
when the analyst interprets at the beginning of the session and
second when there is a long interpretation and the patient
merely says "Yes." It is at this point that the analyst continues
to interpret without allowing room for the patient's experience.

I explore this issue further in the discussion at the end
of this chapter. Clearly, the session presented does not represent predominantly oedipal or object love experiences.

## Case Material: The Independent Analyst

I do not quite agree with the Independent analyst that the
session he reports on is an oedipal session. The more important point, however, is that the treatment seems to have been
life saving for the patient. I also agree with the patient when
she corrects him; he says that "I'm the instructor who helped
you to swim." She says to him, "I don't think you ever instructed me, or showed me how to do anything. I feel you
are the water."

In this session the Independent analyst provided the
space for the patient, Mrs. T., to display and look at her pro-

tective omnipotence and allowed her masochism and sadness to be contained mostly within the treatment. He showed the flexibility to allow her to beat him to the punch (with the answers or interpretations). The main issue was not a phallic rivalry fueled by hostility to men. She was attempting to demonstrate that, if need be, she could survive without men or without an omniscient parent. She knew all the answers. It seems as if he gently but firmly "corrected her" or gave his contrary interpretations, which helped her begin to feel she could survive in the water (go on being) even if at times her strokes were not the smoothest. In the session she puts together different aspects of the analyst and is able simultaneously to tolerate both her wishes to destroy him and her idealization of him. She is clearly better able at the end of treatment to tolerate her envy of the powerful male figure, and she and the analyst have untangled some of the roots of her powerful masochistic identifications. She has been able to tolerate the narcissistic humiliations that have plagued her for her entire life. She has become active and autonomous, finally leaving her crippling and I suspect crippled husband, and is willing to now become more fully alive. The questions for her were preoedipal questions, and her life was in one way dominated by its traumatic beginnings.

## Concluding Comments

The movement away from larger theoretical statements is embedded in the Freudian analyst's comment that in Britain today we tend to focus on "transference manifestations in the here and now of the session." However, her interpretations contained both transference and reconstructive elements. Moreover, they depended on particular theoretical ideas about childhood conflicts and the infantile neurosis. The concept of the here-and-now transference is a redundant one, since the theory of transference necessarily implies activity in the present. I have previously critiqued Gill's ideas about the here-and-now transference (Ellman 1991), but for the purposes of this chapter I comment on only one aspect of this idea. The notion of the here-and-now transference is useful only as a heuristic device. It is a reminder of how easy it is to circumvent the unfolding of transference reactions in an analysis. Conceptually, little is added to Freud's or Bird's ideas about transference. Moreover, the way the concept has been used takes us away from the essence of psychoanalysis, i.e., unconscious fantasy. It also seems to suggest a type of pseudo-empiricism that has gained some popularity in psychoanalysis. It is as if we are not dependent on our theoretical concepts in the clinical situation. It is interesting to note that all of the British analysts seemed to freely use interpretations that depend on reconstructions.

Many of my comments have focused on whether or not the patients that were presented function primarily on an oedipal level. One could well ask whether it really matters. What would one do differently if one were certain that a patient was in fact functioning on a preoedipal as opposed to an oedipal level? There are several possible answers to the question, but let us first return to Mrs. T., the patient of the Independent analyst. She felt rebuffed by interpretations and frequently was silent for long periods, saying, "I like listening to your breathing; it reassures me that you're alive." Patients such as Mrs. T., during some phases of an analysis, are unable to process interpretive efforts. They might hear your speech pattern, the quality of your voice, but the content of the interpretation is gone. Some patients might simply withdraw or become compliant as a type of withdrawal (Winnicott 1955). Mrs. T is a type of patient frequently described by Kohut (1971), Bach (1985, 1994), and Kernberg (1975). Kohut (1971) recommends that with such a patient one should not interpret at the beginning of the treatment. Bach

has advocated modifications of the Kohutian approach. It is
the beginning of the treatment that is modified in his approach. His views on other phases of analytic treatment are
quite different from Kohut's. Frequently this type of narcissistic character is not able to tolerate interpretations, and
Mrs. T. exhibited one familiar type of response to analytic
interpretations. In an earlier work, I described a patient who
would begin to howl if she sensed that I was about to make
an interpretation (Ellman 1991). Mrs. T. did everything she
could to disrupt the Independent analyst's interpretative
efforts. She attempted to anticipate his responses, and she
seemingly felt crushed when she was unable to prevent his
making an interpretive comment. Patients who have predominantly oedipal conflicts usually do not continuously
display the type of behavior that the Independent analyst
experienced with Mrs. T. The systematic development of
analytic trust (Ellman 1991) is crucial in the treatment of this
type of patient, who in the United States is frequently labeled
a nonclassical patient.

Thus Mrs. T. required a different analytic stance than
did Dr. A., the subject of the Freudian analysis. He was clearly
able to use interpretative efforts, and this was probably true
throughout his treatment with the Freudian analyst. The
establishment of analytic trust occurs virtually unnoticed in
the course of the treatment with many neurotic patients. Two
interrelated factors describe the marked differences between
Mrs. T. and Dr. A.: the establishment of trust in the analytic
situation and their response to interpretations.

It is also possible to look at the Kleinian analyst's approach to this type of patient. Analysts, for periods of time,
should be willing to give up the role of the objective decoder
of meaning. During these periods they should instead allow
themselves to become part of the narcissistically vulnerable
patient's subjective world. The Independent analyst did this,
although at times reluctantly, whereas the Kleinian analyst
attempted to stay in the role of the decoder of meaning. The

tone of the session was set by the latter's interpretations of the patient's internal world. A theory that states the patient's world in objective terms, as does both the Kleinian and classical positions, will tend to position its practitioners in the consistent role of interpreters.

These comments are not meant to denigrate the role of interpretation or insight in the psychoanalytic process. Rather the analyst–patient relationship is more central in some theories than in others. Kohut and intersubjective analysts (Kohut 1982, Stolorow 1991) are at one extreme of this continuum, whereas Kleinian analysts are frequently at the other end. In the United States Ogden is an example of a Kleinian analyst who is attempting to develop concepts that cross this boundary. That the Kleinian analyst in the session she presented is at one end of the interpretive continuum is in part a function of her theoretical stance.[2] Notwithstanding my criticism, the Kleinian and neo-Kleinian theoretical perspective is a rich and important one, one in which I find much of great value.

If I am correct that Dr. A. is the only oedipal patient who has been presented, one might wonder why this is the case. It seems likely to me that both the Independent and Kleinian analysts are aware that their patients' primary difficulties were not oedipal in nature. It could be that either or both of the authors chose the cases they did for trivial reasons, i.e., this was the easiest case to write up or they had no better examples of oedipal sessions at this particular point in time. In part it is the theories they adhere to that made

---

2. Clearly the Kleinian analyst was able to empathically capture the patient's world by the end of the session she presented. This is a good argument for convergence in psychoanalysis. Even though I believe she interpreted far too freely, her obvious analytic tact and sensitivity made such technical reservations somewhat beside the point. Thus it is clear that a good clinician utilizing any theoretical vantage point will be effective.

the issue less important than it would be for a Freudian analyst. If a main focus of one's theory is to differentiate between positions (paranoid-schizoid and depressive) or to look at the psychotic versus the nonpsychotic aspects of the personality, then oedipal dynamics may not be terribly important. Similarly, if one sees oedipal dynamics coursing through the developmental cycle, the questions I have raised may seem quite unimportant. However, if the issue of analyzability rests on whether or not the patient has primarily oedipal conflicts, then obviously this concern becomes greatly magnified. In addition, if your theory at one point avowed the centrality of the oedipal phase (Freudian thought after the structural model), then this theoretical stance obviously colors your view of the significance of oedipal factors.

It is my conclusion that theoretical orientation played a part in the selection of the patient and in how each of the analysts conducted his or her session. However, none of the authors has fully spelled out his or her theoretical orientation, and so one might say that I am piling inference upon inference. As a more general point, theoretical positions today are far less certain than they seemed to be thirty years ago. Is Ogden (1991, a representative of a Kleinian position, or do we have to rely on Segal (1983, 1987) in the British school for a truly neo-Kleinian perspective? Clearly we have to wait to evaluate the integrative concepts that Ogden is trying to develop to answer this question more fully. In a similar vein one can ask whether Bach (1985, 1994) is a true representation of contemporary Freudian thought, or do we have to rely on Brenner (1987) to define a genuine Freudian analyst? Lipton has even questioned (1977, 1979) whether we should equate classical analysts with the term *Freudian* analysts. Bach's attempts to include a self perspective within a Freudian approach might seem to some an inappropriate mixture of theoretical models. To others it may seem to be a solution to some questions that have long vexed Freudian clinicians.

Ogden and Bach are clinicians who are attempting integrations across theoretical boundaries. They are doing this, however, not by polemic or assertion but rather by developing concepts that attempt to explain clinical phenomena. They also include implicit rules of correspondence within their theoretical purviews. For example, in Bach's work the patient's ability to tolerate multiple perspectives provides a theoretical anchor that allows one to draw inferences that directly relate to psychoanalytic technique. This and other concepts that he develops allow the clinician to have a point of reference in determining what he believes will and will not succeed in clinical work with various patient populations.

In this chapter I have maintained that theoretical perspectives assert both implicit and explicit effects on how an analyst behaves in the clinical situation. I have also proposed that, until we understand the extent of this influence more fully, it will be difficult to undertake meaningful integrations. If this book had been written thirty years ago, my assertions would have been considered quite unnecessary. At that time everyone knew that theory strictly determined an analyst's behavior. We seem to have advanced a good deal in questioning our assumptions about the relationship of theory to clinical practice. In a small way I have endeavored to show that an influence we once assumed was profound is still present in at least subtler forms. Moreover, it may be that the integration and common ground that many analysts are searching for can be found only when they have explored and understood the terrain they have once inhabited.

## References

Abelin, E. L. (1975). Some further observations and comments on the earliest role of the father. *International Journal of Psycho-Analysis* 56(3):293–302.

Bach, S. (1985). *Narcissistic States and the Therapeutic Process.*
    Northvale, NJ: Jason Aronson.
——— (1994). *The Language of Perversion and the Language of
    Love.* Northvale, NJ: Jason Aronson.
Bird, B. (1972). Notes on transference: universal phenom-
    enon and hardest part of analysis. *Journal of the Ameri-
    can Psychoanalytic Association* 20(2):267–301.
Brenner, C. (1987). How theory shapes technique: perspec-
    tives on a clinical study: a structural theory perspective.
    *Psychoanalytic Inquiry* 7(2):167–171.
Ellman, S. J. (1991). *Freud's Technique Papers.* Northvale, NJ:
    Jason Aronson.
Freud, A. (1936). *The Ego and Mechanisms of Defence.* New
    York: International Universities Press.
Freud, S. (1910). Leonardo da Vinci and a memory of his
    childhood. *Standard Edition* 2:59–137.
——— (1911). Psycho-analytic notes on an autobiographical
    account of a case of paranoia (dementia paranoides).
    *Standard Edition* 12:9–82.
——— (1913). The disposition to obsessional neurosis: a con-
    tribution to the problem of choice of neurosis. *Standard
    Edition* 12:317–326.
——— (1914). On narcissism: an introduction. *Standard Edi-
    tion* 14:73–102.
——— (1915). Papers on metapsychology: instincts and their
    vicissitudes. *Standard Edition* 14:117–140.
——— (1917). Papers on metapsychology: mourning and mel-
    ancholia [1915]. *Standard Edition* 14:237–258.
Jacobson, E. (1954). The self and the object world. *Psycho-
    analytic Study of the Child* 9:75–127.
——— (1964). *The Self and the Object World.* New York: Inter-
    national Universities Press.
Kernberg, O. (1975). *Borderline Conditions and Pathological
    Narcissism.* New York: Jason Aronson.

Kohut, H. (1971). *The Analysis of the Self.* New York: International Universities Press.

—— (1982). Introspection, empathy, and the semi-circle of mental health. *International Journal of Psycho-Analysis* 63(4):395–407.

Lipton S. D. (1977). The advantages of Freud's technique as shown in his analysis of the Rat Man. *International Journal of Psycho-Analysis* 58:255–274.

—— (1979). An addendum to "The Advantages of Freud's Technique as Shown in the Analysis of the Rat Man." *International Journal of Psycho-Analysis* 60:215–216.

Mahler, M. S., Pine, F., and Bergman, A. (1975). *The Psychological Birth of the Human Infant.* New York: Basic Books.

Ogden, T. H. (1991). Analysing the matrix of transference. *International Journal of Psycho-Analysis* 72(4):593–605.

Pine, F. (1988). The four psychologies of psychoanalysis and their place in clinical work. *Journal of the American Psychoanalytic Association* 36(3):571–596.

Reed, G. S. (1990). A reconsideration of the concept of transference neurosis. *International Journal of Psycho-Analysis* 71(2):205–217.

Sandler, J. (1983). Discussions with Anna Freud on *The Ego and the Mechanisms of Defence: The Ego and the Id at Puberty. International Journal of Psycho-Analysis* 64(4):401–406.

Sandler, J., and Sandler, A.-M. (1983). The 'second censorship,' the 'three box model' and some technical implications. *International Journal of Psycho-Analysis* 64(4):413–425.

—— (1984). The past unconscious, the present unconscious, and interpretation of the transference [Commentary on Merton Gill's "Analysis of Transference"]. *Psychoanalytic Inquiry* 4(3):367–399.

—— (1994). *Comments on the conceptualization of clinical facts*

*in psychoanalysis. Presented at the 75th Anniversary Celebra-
tion of International Journal of Psychoanalysis,* Westpoint,
N. Y.

Segal, H. (1983). Some clinical implications of Melanie Klein's
work. Emergence from narcissism. *International Journal
of Psycho-Analysis* 64(3):269–280.

—— (1987). Silence is the real crime. *International Review of
Psycho-Analysis* 14(1):3–12.

Stolorow, R. D. (1991). The intersubjective context of intrapsychic experience: a decade of psychoanalytic inquiry.
*Psychoanalytic Inquiry* 11(1–2):171–184.

Wallerstein, R. S. (1990). Psychoanalysis: the common ground.
*International Journal of Psycho-Analysis* 71(1):3–20.

Winnicott, D. W. (1955). Metapsychologic and clinical aspects
of regression within the psycho-analytical set-up. *International Journal of Psycho-Analysis* 36(1):16–26.

# 7

## Commentary by Fred Pine

Chapters 3 through 5 presented three very different sessions from three very experienced analysts. Each session reflects a patient–analyst pair that is used to working together; they know each other well.

In this chapter I do not attempt to reinterpret the sessions or offer additional interventions. The analysts are experienced; the sessions seem convincing, each in its own way; and I assume that the analysts have a long history, including other material regarding their patients, that leads them to choose the general line of interpretation, or the specific form of interpretation, that they follow. I therefore give a sympathetic reading of the sessions.

In this chapter, I examine the three sessions individually and comparatively to discuss issues of technique, as embodied in these three sets of process notes. In this exploration I focus on the analysts, not the patients. Of course, two questions are built into the very structure of the study. The first question—embodied in the selection of the three speakers from the British Kleinian, Freudian (the "modern" or "contemporary" Kleinian and Freudian), and Independent groups—is, Can we see differences in theory or technique among the groups? The second question—stemming from the instruction to the three to report a session in which oedipal content is central—has to do with our current understanding or *their* understanding of that concept today.

In answer to the first question of whether there are differences in theory and technique among the presentations, I—an American—hearing them for the first time and trying to look at them like a naive observer—would argue that it is not possible to clearly separate out differences that stem from multiple sources: theoretical differences and differences in individual style *perhaps,* but also certainly patient differences, differences in the context of particular sessions, and (related to context) differences having to do with the timing of a session, its place in the course of the analysis.

I discuss the three presentations in the order in which I received them because that reflects the way my thoughts developed as I went from one to the next to the next.

### The Kleinian Analysis

The Kleinian analyst's patient has just come back from vacation, and the office had been redecorated in her absence. She missed a session, had trouble getting to another one because of traffic, and then her analyst was three minutes late for the session that is reported here. The tone of the session is set in the first three things the analyst tells us:

> I kept her waiting three minutes. She lay down and spoke about the traffic: it was absolutely horrible today! She doesn't understand it; whichever way she tries to get here there is traffic and it's blocked up, difficult. She tried to take a new route—but once she got round the corner it was completely blocked up.
>
> I knew she was talking about a real, external event, but I felt sure she was also speaking about her response to being kept waiting.

I said that I thought my keeping her waiting this morning was horrible for her, that she feels that there has been some kind of traffic in this room that has blocked up her access to me and made her feel how really difficult she feels it is to actually get back to me.

This intervention sets the tone. In fact, the Kleinian analyst's interpretations are heavily, though by no means completely, of the form: "You are talking about you and me." This can become clear by examining *all* of her interventions:

1. I said that I thought my keeping her waiting this morning was horrible for her. That she feels that there has been some kind of traffic in this room that has blocked up her access to me and made her feel how really difficult she feels it is to actually get back to me.

2. I said I thought she had been trying to tell me how she feels, but that something then had come along inside her and interfered.

3. I said that when I was late today it made her feel that something—some*one* was keeping me away from her—was interfering with her getting to me. I thought *that* was what was hurting her and that she experienced it not so much in her feelings as in her arm. And I thought that when she came into the room and became aware of its being redecorated, it hit her with a bang—that someone else has been with me, inside of me, occupying me and doing things with and to me while she had to wait.

4. I said that I thought that when she was in the waiting room and when she'd come into the room she felt very much the way she described feeling when she was a little girl. I think she wants to mess me up, like smearing the wallpaper and messing the bed, partly because she's angry with me, but mostly because she would much rather imagine her*self* as the messer-upper, the main person, than to feel as left out as she feels when she thinks someone else is here with me, "messing me up." I said I thought when she feels someone else is with me it makes her feel impossibly left out and jealous.

5. I said I think it feels terrible for her to feel like the little girl at the end of the corridor, or in the waiting room. I said I think that, when that happens, she switches things around in her mind—she imagines herself as the "Daddy"—the one who gets to be with the "Mummy."

6. I said I thought the affair with the student in her dream felt like a love affair with me, but without sexuality and without jealousy and therefore without the messing up that makes her feel so heavy and bad inside. I said that I thought in this dream, with a student connected to me, with me in the background, she has created or found the "tube" that would enable us to be sexless but perfect lovers. I spoke about her feelings as a little girl of not having a penis and therefore having to invent a "tube" that would enable her to be close to her mother in the way she wanted. I suggested that in this dream she had created a relationship to me which made her terribly happy, which was not spoiled by the presence of a father, and therefore

one in which jealousy is left out. I thought this got rid of the pain of jealousy from her mind—and therefore from her arm.

7. I said that the dream seemed to offer a cure for that sadness [sadness that "my analyst will never really love me"]—no wonder she wanted so much to hold onto it in the night.

These are mostly, though not entirely, of the sort "you are talking about you and me." But of course the analyst is listening to her patient—and *what* she says the patient is saying with respect to the analyst keeps expanding and modifying in accord with the patient's associations.

Today, we all tend to value work in the here and now, the "you are talking about you and me" approach. Wrongly used, however, this approach has its dangers—perhaps the creation of a dual solipsism in which the patient's history and world no longer matter or perhaps excessive gratification in the intensity of the relationship. For both therapist and patient, this gratification may itself become a collusive enactment. But the Kleinian analyst's reported session certainly does not seem to fall into these dangers, and indeed she continually draws on the patient's associations about her world to redefine what is happening "here" in the session. The advantage of the here-and-now approach is clear: it produces much greater immediacy and affective intensity in the work. In my experience, not all patients allow you to achieve such immediacy because something about their associative style or general character blocks it or rebels against it. The late emergence of the dream from the night before—regarding her crush on the student—and the associations to its having begun at the Christmas break from analysis lend strong support to the analyst's sense that the separation issue between patient and herself was paramount, even when ex-

pressed in terms of distance from the parental bedroom and
masturbation, that is, the patient's occupying herself while
alone. But, and here is why I am unable to draw any conclusions about the Kleinian style or group differences from this
session, there is a very strong determinative *context* for this
session: it is after a vacation and the analyst is late. It is like
a session presurgery or after the death of a parent in which
the analyst feels he or she knows what the content is *likely* to
be about. And this particular content (in the analyst's eyes,
and I see no reason to disagree) *is* about "you're talking about
me", i.e., *is* about the separation and the lateness and the
patient's response to it. The analyst keeps showing her that
her feelings and her associations are expanding on that
central theme.

## The Independent Analysis

The session presented by the Independent analyst is very
different. The patient had a tragic early history with an ill
father and a preoccupied mother. She was mainly very sad.
The patient begins the session with her glee (though it is
short-lived) regarding a supposed "failure" of her analyst in
a long-ago consultation.

    The Independent analyst's interventions, in sharp con-
trast to those of the Kleinian analyst, largely, though by no
means entirely, take the patient out of the room, often to
the past. Ten interventions are reported; they are all brief.

1. To the past: "You have a need for idols, but
   you find it exciting when they fall, as Father
   did."
2. The past and the inside present: the patient
   had just said that she was a head-banger as a
   child, perhaps in identification with Father's

"turns." "And if I 'fall' by being a useless consultant, I seem to be the father, always liable to fall."

3. The inside present: "So you felt you could tell me about my useless consultation without fearing I would be in tears."

4. The inside present: "You are reassuring me now, but also managing to say, 'We are all the same.'"

5. The past: "I think your search for weakness in men (husband, father, me) is not only a wish to triumph but also to find a weak father to at last replace Mother, and you can look after the weak father."

6. The past: "You probably also believed it was you, by your birth, or your badness who caused his illness."

7. The past and the inside present: "Today, you show how much you need to make me the father who is knocked down (the bad consultation), but then also, quickly revived (by reporting the good consultation)."

8. The outside present: "I think you are saying you have accepted that your marriage is at an end."

9. The inside present: "Perhaps you are saying, 'Haven't we done well to avoid change?'"

10. The inside present: "I'm the instructor who helped you to swim."

Why the relatively larger focus on the past? It may be the Independent analyst's regular way of working, but I see two other possible reasons for it here. The first is that in contrast to the Kleinian analyst's patient, this patient is talking explicitly about the analyst. This material could have been explored further within itself, even by simply inviting a closer description about the patient's experience. But the Independent analyst does what we commonly do: he goes to a domain different from but parallel to the patient's—that is, he roves among transference, the outside present, and the past—to show links and repetitions.

The second, more individualized, reason for bringing things to the past here has to do with *context* again. And here the context is *termination.* And, from the patient's continued struggle with the analyst at this late point and her saying, "One line I recall was 'Don't hope to arise from the dead'," (for the analyst tells us: "She identified with a very morose father, lacking spontaneity, and she was herself internally dead, always completely anorgasmic, and terrified that sexual excitement stood for, or could provoke, a seizure"), I read it as a termination in a patient who, not surprisingly, continues to live much of her tragic history in her current life. "Deadness," or the fear of full engagement with people who will fall, die, abandon, or make her feel dead again, is built into her deeply. From the outside, one can wonder, Could more have been done? Could the dead self have been approached more fully? But the experience of working with severely developmentally traumatized patients teaches us respect for limits. Psychoanalysis *has* its limits. I am sure the Independent analyst feels much was approached, reached, and even altered—and I do not doubt that.

However, there is one reported intervention that seems like a real sidestepping of the patient's thoughts. She says about a funeral she attended, "I'd like that kind of funeral for me. One line I recall was 'Don't hope to arise from the dead.'" The analyst responds, "I think you are saying you have accepted that your marriage is at an end." She seems to be saying a lot more than that, although I cannot from the outside say what most needed response.

Despite the fact that the Independent analyst quotes

Ernst Ticho regarding no changes in technique at termination, the analyst is trying to give this damaged woman, now close to termination, as full a grasp as possible of the continued impact of her past story, to give her maximal control over its effects upon her now. He is choosing then—near termination—*not* to say (primarily), "This is what is happening between us," but instead to say (more often), "This is what we've learned together; this is my parting gift to you." In addition, by his tone of speaking, he seems to be conveying empathically, his understanding of the tragedy of her life.

## The Freudian Analysis

The patient of the Freudian analyst was the man who saw her husband and his patient in the waiting room, had ejaculated during fellatio the night before, had been promoted over his colleague's head, and brought in material suggestive of shame over being caught in his sexual looking and of feared retaliation for his victories.

This analyst's interventions are fewer, though one is quite long, and they come much later in the session—the first apparently after about half the time had elapsed. In contrast, both the Independent and Kleinian analysts had spoken much earlier on.

The Freudian analyst writes at the outset, "My own technical approach, which, although rooted in developmental thinking, gives *priority* to the analysis of the 'here and now,' with reconstruction in terms of the specific patient's development being used to provide a temporal dimension to the patient's insight." And that is indeed what she seems to do. She addresses what is going on and, in her final comment, "provides a temporal dimension"—the role of the past. Here are her four interventions:

1. Accordingly, I limited myself to saying, "When I think of your dream, and what happened with Stephanie last night, I cannot help but feel that in your mind Stephanie, your mother, and I were all mixed up."

2. "On Friday you told me that you were very pleased with the way our work was going. You told me of the promotion you had been offered and that you felt how much you had changed because of our analytic work. I think that these feelings made you rather scared and that you became afraid that my husband would resent the fact that you and I were getting on so well."

3. I commented, "Perhaps there is a part of you that would like to have my husband out of the way so that you can have me all to yourself. But I think that this makes you uneasy, and so you feel the need to make your peace with him, too."

4. The longer final intervention: I remarked, "You must have been terribly frightened then, and I think that when you say you looked at the scar you must also have been checking up on your 'willy' [the patient's word for his penis] to see if it was still there. I think thoughts about Jack's operation and your own came to your mind just now because of a fear that my husband would revenge himself for your excitement about his female patient and about me, that he would punish and emasculate you for daring to want him out of the way. But I think that all of this has been triggered by your promotion—you've been more successful than your father was, and we know that you have been very guilty about that. We also know that you are aware of the fact that you can allow yourself to do better

because of our work here, but it scares you. It
is as if you take my husband's women away from
him—his patient and me, and in the past your
father's woman—your mother. So you expect
punishment."

In contrast to the Kleinian and Independent analyst's
patients where a context for the session was clearly present
(postseparation and pretermination, respectively), the context with this patient was not clear until the session was well
under way—that context ultimately coming to be seen as his
promotion over his colleague's head and his expressed feelings of pleasure to his analyst in the previous session that his
and her work together was going well. This was what he had
come in with—in his head and apparently on his shoulders.

The Freudian analyst writes that before her first intervention she wanted to delay intervention and to find an
emotionally convincing way to intervene in light of her
patient's tendency to intellectualize—and her first three interventions clearly are meant to stir the emotional pot just a
bit. She also writes that this oedipal material was new, that
"it had not been much in evidence in the analysis before."
Taking into account all of these statements, as well as her
writing at the start that the task of finding an oedipal session
for presentation was "far from easy," I began to wonder
whether this presentation was on the analyst's shoulders at
some point in this session. Nonetheless, the material is indeed very convincing on the oedipal theme: memories of his
mother's nonpunishment contrasting to his father's insistence on it, being "caught" by the analyst's husband (and his
father in the past) at voyeuristic activity, competition, victory,
and the like.

Long interventions are not foreign to my way of working. Every analysis needs an "aria" by the analyst now and
then. It can pull things together. And the patient needs to

hear the analyst's voice, even simply resaying what the patient already knows. But as the danger in here-and-now "you're talking about me" interventions can be solipsism or enactment (whereas the gain is immediacy), the danger in long interconnecting interventions such as the Freudian analyst's final one, or in reconstructive interventions, like some of the Independent analyst's, is overload or intellectualization. The gain in them is clearly *understanding*. Evolution gave us feelings that act as signals and a mind that can understand. I do not give *experiencing* pride of place over understanding in psychoanalysis. They both matter. And they do not ordinarily conflict, because understanding in the transference usually guarantees simultaneous experiencing. But both experiencing and understanding can become resistances, can clog up the process. I wish we knew how and whether the Freudian analyst's patient was able to use that end-of-session interpretation, but the session ended there.

### Are There Differences Among the Groups?

Perhaps I am being too integrative, eclectic, or ecumenical—and, if so, it wouldn't be the first time—but I find nothing in these three presentations that permits me to separate out group differences. None of the presentations seemed particularly theory-driven; each seemed to reveal the responsiveness of the analyst to what the patient brought in. The inferential leaps from the content were not large (I say this in a positive sense), but stayed close to what seemed to be the patient's clinical issues. There *are* differences in the locale of the interventions—between patient and analyst, to the past, and movement between these domains—but they are relative, not absolute. Furthermore, all of the forms of intervention seem to sit comfortably within what we regard as reasonably familiar psychoanalytic technique. They certainly used forms of intervention that I use every day, and I do not find myself feeling part of different groups as I use them. In fact, the differences seem at least in substantial part to reflect differences in the patients, in what I have called the context of the session (when in the analysis it is happening) and the particular content that the patient has brought in. There *are* substantial differences in these sessions, but they seem no more different than the differences might be among any single analyst's first three sessions of the day. There is, of course, no basis for making large pronouncements about the three British groups from this small sample of data. However, if these sessions reflect ways that these three analysts work *regularly* and if their within-group colleagues do the same, then I would argue that there *are* group differences along immediacy/distance or experiencing/understanding dimensions. But I would add that there *shouldn't* be such differences because any one way is too limiting.

From this brief review of the three presentations, I want to discuss two general issues in the theory of psychoanalytic technique in the 1990s, *our* "here and now": interpretation in the here and now of the transference and one-person and two-person psychologies.

## Interpretations in the
## Here and Now of the Transference

The phrase, "interpretations in the here and now of the transference" has at least three differentiable meanings: First, from the outside into the office: "You think you are talking about something out there, but it is really about me (or about us)." This in contrast to Freud's earliest discovery about transference, which goes, "What you think you are feeling or imagining about me is really about person X from your past." Interpretation from the outside in ("it's really about me or

us") seems clearly linked to Gill's (1982) idea of first interpreting resistance to the *awareness* of transference, that is,
by showing the patient that there are transference manifestations in many places. Second, the here-and-now transference is worked with because it is brought in by some patients
who often, or even regularly, come in and talk about the
analyst and their relation to him or her. These are patients
who might seem to the uninitiated to be curable by leaving
the analysis; all of their problems seem to be with the analyst or the analysis. The analyst works with this here and now
presumably with the underlying idea that the analytic events
are a microcosm of the patient's world and that therefore
the work is properly done within the analysis. And third, the
here and now of the transference refers to enactments: "It's
not what you are *saying* here that counts (at this moment)
because what's really important is what is *happening between
us,* a something that you are living out—in your mood, your
way of speaking, the atmosphere you set up, the way you
entrap me into being, and so on." This last point—the
patient's getting the analyst to be, do, or feel a certain way—
is talked about as an induced effect and often as projective
identification. I still find that term to be too omni-meaninged
—that is, it seems to mean too many things—and, in fact, I
am totally uncertain about the Kleinian analyst's usage of it
when she writes at the end of the chapter, "Instead of feeling herself to be the little girl pushed out by a father who
is doing things to Mother, she has, by means of projective
identification, become the father." Why not just the word
"identification" there? In these presentations, of the three
forms of the here and now, we read a lot about the first (bringing the outside to the inside), some about the second (patient speaking directly of his or her involvement with the
analyst, which then becomes a focus), and little of the third
(enactments).

## One- or Two-Person Psychologies

Clearly, the three presentations focused on one-person psychology. They were dominated by the analyst as expert telling the patient what was going on *in the patient*–whether or not what was going on was related to the analyst. It was all *in* the patient. The free association instruction and the couch tilt things in this direction. They say: "You are the specimen; move around under my microscope for a while until I can see what you are doing, and then I'll tell you." One might think that a long delay before the first intervention, as in the Freudian analyst's case, might heighten this tendency, but it is clear that even the much earlier interventions by the Kleinian and Independent analysts are along the same line. They simply say: "I have figured out what you are doing more quickly, so I'll tell you now." I generally work this way (i.e., within a one-person psychology), although I try to be alert to my place in the process. Others surely work much more in a two-person psychology way. Theories of technique and personal style enter in heavily here, and no doubt a convinced two-person psychologist could translate these three presentations into those terms. For some patients–some of mine certainly–the work goes in that direction in a major way. Some patients, free association and the couch notwithstanding, force a two-person psychoanalysis by their way of being, by the enactments they draw the analyst into, by their capacity to see inside the analyst and make his or her way of being, and the patient's experience of that being a focus of the work. Therefore, the one-person/two-person issue is also in substantial part reflective of patient differences, not only the technical or theoretical preferences of analysts (though that also). Both ways of working should therefore be available to all analysts. The couch nicely places the patient midway between being *alone* and being *with* someone. And each state is a significant part of psychic functioning, even if alone states involve that patient with internal objects. The patient can turn inward or outward, and that choice itself reflects the patient's psychology of the moment.

If the Independent analyst had chosen to work actively with whatever it was in his patient that led him to attempt to keep to a "strictly disciplined technique" with her and would have allowed himself to do instead whatever it was that he might usually do, and to work with the patient's *experience* of this, we would have had an instance of a two-person psychology at work. I suppose we *did* have that, actually, but it took the form of the disciplined technique and the patient's seeming to require it and prefer it, instead of its being a subject of the analysis.

### The Oedipal Content of the Presentations

The study format itself raised two issues—first, the comparison of the three British groups (which I have chosen to view by way of three analysts and their three individual patients at three different moments in their analyses, rather than as representatives of groups); and second, the instruction to bring in a session with oedipal content.

The Kleinian analyst presents a patient who goes associatively from a separation and a lateness to being "down a long corridor" from the parental bedroom, but she believes the central issue for the patient is the *separation from the analyst,* who, in the analyst's formulation, is imagined to have other people with her—oedipal-like. That is, she sees the possibly triangular content as revealing (in this particular session) what the patient does when alone—masturbating, messing, attempting to be the *active* one. And the Independent analyst presents a patient who, in his formulation, wants to build up and care for a father better than her mother did, but the tragic early history of the patient makes clear that the central formative issues long precede oedipal fantasies— indeed they begin to take shape before her birth when the father's life changed. And the Freudian analyst, who clearly does focus on more developmentally advanced, oedipal, triangular, sexually rivalrous issues in this particular session, writes that these issues had been absent from the analysis until then and indeed that it was "far from easy" to find an oedipal session in her practice altogether.

I attended the first World Congress of Infant Psychiatry in 1980 where much research on the "competent infant" was presented. Erik Erikson was invited to make a few summary comments at the end; after hearing all of the reports of cognitive-perceptual-relational research on infancy, he began by asking, plaintively, "Whatever happened to the oral phase?"! So after reading these presentations, we might ask, though not plaintively: What is happening to the oedipal phase? Imagine how absent it might have been if the editors had not specifically asked for oedipal content.

The oedipal phase and oedipal fantasy and wishes are very much present, but they are not the full story and often not the main story. Oedipal fantasies (triangular—the child's relation to two parents) may give shape to all that has gone before, but so does all that has gone before force a particular shape or quality on the oedipal constellation. It is like building a house. The house may look like a house, though the construction may be of straw or mud or bricks. That is, the constituent elements of the oedipal situation (the earlier developmental history) vary enormously, and the oedipal can only be what the early constituents (the straw or mud or bricks) allow it to be. And some of the building blocks may be defective (ego defects), and some may be missing (deficits). And there may be special building blocks that totally color everything about the oedipal situation— for example, if all the building blocks are painted black by chronic mood states such as "deadness."

These presentations are not unique. With a century now of clinical observation and the expansion of theory, and decades of analytically sophisticated infant and child observation, we have a far more sophisticated view of early development and its expression in psychopathology. Or perhaps—in an age of theoretical uncertainty—we can simply listen more openly and hear things in more diverse ways.

Have I minimized the differences among the British groups? Do they not show up as dramatically in these presentations as they might? And if I have failed to see them as clearly as I might have, what are they? Or are between-patient differences and between-individual–analyst differences larger than any group commonalities? Or, again, is it all in flux, or obscure, or do presentations on divergent theories make differences look larger than day-to-day working sessions actually demonstrate? Please educate us.

## Reference

Gill, M. M. (1982). *Analysis of Transference. Vol. I. Theory and Technique.* New York: International Universities Press.

# 8

# Commentary by
# Robert Wallerstein:
# Common Ground or Not?

In my plenary addresses to the International Psycho-Analytical Association Congress in Montreal in 1987 (Wallerstein 1988) and to the following Congress in Rome in 1989 (Wallerstein 1990) I developed two interlocked themes: (1) the issue created for psychoanalysis as a science and a discipline by the increasing acknowledgment and acceptance of the diversity (or pluralism) of psychoanalytic theoretical perspectives that had developed since Freud's day and (2) what in the face of this diversity has held us all together as psychoanalysts—where was our common ground? The overall thesis that I developed in those addresses can be stated in summary form. It is that our growing theoretical diversification within psychoanalysis, going back as far as the growth of the Kleinian movement in the 1920s and still in Freud's active lifetime, has represented a diversity of conceptual explanatory systems (general psychologies, metapsychologies) devised to best explain—for their adherents—the *common* clinical phenomena of conflict and its compromise, anxiety and symptoms, defense and resistance, and transference and countertransference. These phenomena are common in both senses of being the usual, ordinary phenomena with which all practicing psychoanalysts deal in their day-to-day work in their consulting rooms and in the sense of being shared as the common data—what we consider to be the observables in our work, whatever our metapsychological theoretical allegiances. That is, our diversity exists in our experience-distant *general theories,* our theoretical explanatory systems created to give coherence and order and a sense of overall understanding—psychological understanding in terms of a theory of mind and mental functioning—to the phenomena observed in the consulting room; our common ground exists in our experience-near *clinical theory* encompassing the discernible clinical events of conflict, resistance, and transference–countertransference interplay palpable in our daily clinical encounters.

To me, the clinical theory, being grounded in observables, is amenable then to the selfsame processes of hypothesis formation, testing, and validation as any other scientific enterprise, albeit, of course, by methods adapted to the peculiar subjectivistic nature of the essential data from the psychoanalytic situation. The general theories—our diverse metapsychologies, the ego psychological, Kleinian, object-relational, self psychological, interpersonal, Lacanian, Bionian, and so on—I see, at least at this stage of our historic developmental dynamic, as primarily metaphoric, our large-scale explanatory metaphors, or symbolisms that we use to give a sense of coherence and closure to our psychological understandings and therefore to our psychoanalytic interventions. They are therefore our pluralistic psychoanalytic articles of faith that I feel in our current developmental state to be essentially beyond the realm of empirical study and scientific process.

Clearly my argument rests on the relative distance between the general theories—the ego psychological theory of id, ego, and superego and their interrelationships; the Kleinian theory of part and whole objects and of paranoid and depressive positions; the self psychological theory of the bipolar self with its twin poles of ambitions and of values adhered to, connected by a "tension arc" of talents and capacities; and the object relational theory of self and object representations and the emotional valences that link them—and the clinical phenomena and clinical theories and the fact that we have no established canons of inference to help or guide the inferential leap from the level of clinical theory to that of general theory. This speaks of course to the conception of a relative disjunction between theory (general theory) and technique (the application of the concepts of the clinical theory) and a putative connection between the two levels that at its (inferential) best is elastic indeed.

As is pointed out in this book by Daniel Hill, many disagree with the notion of so significant a disjuncture between theory and technique; they feel that there is a more significant determining imprint of theory—whether ego psychological, Kleinian, or whatever—upon technique. As a corollary they feel that the common ground I have been pointing to is more illusory than real and that the elements of shared clinical theory I have focused on—conflict, resistance, transference–countertransference, and so on—though carrying the same names, contain enough different meanings, because they are inevitably infiltrated by differing theory-drenched connotations, that they ineluctably lead to consistently different theory-driven technical interventions. Therefore, in fact no such assumed common clinical ground actually exists. The proof of this particular pudding lies of course significantly in the (clinical) eating, and I tried in earlier presentations (Wallerstein 1988, 1990), to give convincing clinical demonstration of my viewpoint.

For my Montreal presentation in 1987 I drew on a clinical vignette reported by Kohut in which he recounted an interchange with a Kleinian colleague from Latin America who told him how she had responded interpretively, in a typically Kleinian format, to a patient's silent withdrawal from the analytic work in the hour immediately after being notified of the planned cancellation of a session in the near future. Kohut, in his account, expressed surprise that this to him "far-fetched interpretation" nonetheless elicited a very favorable response from the patient. Kohut then went on to offer an equally plausible interpretation couched in his own self psychological terms as well as one within ego psychological conflict-defense terms. For Kohut the clinical context given by his Kleinian colleague was insufficient to decide which interpretation would be closest to the mark in this instance and so he called all three of them potential examples of "wild analysis," until proven otherwise. What I made of this account was quite different. I asserted that all three analysts, using differing theoretical explanatory languages, which clearly in Kohut's example were readily identifiable as Kleinian, self psychological, and ego psychological, were nonetheless all centered on a shared clinical meaning— common to all three possible theoretical explanatory languages presented—that the patient was acutely distressed over the impending cancellation and was reacting unhappily and resentfully to that announcement. Given this interpretation of the patient's state of mind and of the perceived meaning of the various analytic responses, the patient could have responded equally favorably to the formulated intervention of whichever of the three postulated analysts (of the three different theoretical perspectives) had been the treating analyst.

The clinical demonstration that I drew on in my Rome presentation in 1989 was the sequence of three main plenary clinical presentations of that Congress representing three major theoretical perspectives in psychoanalysis and the three major worldwide regions of psychoanalytic activity. Anton Kris of Boston presented a paper within the ego psychological (Freudian) framework; Michael Feldman of London presented one within the Kleinian framework; and Max Hernandez of Peru, trained with the Middle or Independent group in London, presented his paper within the object relational framework. These three analysts from three different regions and representing three differing theoretical orientations independently selected three patients, all women within a close age range, who by chance had very much in common, in their personality structures and in their illness pictures, when they came to treatment. In detailed discussion of the three clinical presentations, I concluded that these three analysts, representing the three major regions of worldwide psychoanalytic activity, and trained within three of the major theoretical perspectives within psychoanalysis

> have all approached, dealt with, and interpreted the clinical material of three surprisingly similar and quite comparable analytic patients in a clearly identifiably, and contrary perhaps to our preconceptions, surprisingly comparable way. They have each addressed in quite comparable fashion the phenomena of conflict and compromise, of impulse and defense, of inner and outer object world, of reality and fantasy, of uncovering interpretation and of necessary supportive intervention, i.e., all the interactions within the transference–countertransference matrix that occupy the domain designated by the Sandlers as the "present unconscious." [Wallerstein 1990, p. 18]

The task I have agreed to in connection with this study is exactly comparable to the one I undertook in Rome: to analyze side by side, the clinical presentations of three colleagues, in this instance all from the British Psycho-Analytical Society and representing its three main theoretical positions, now called the Contemporary Freudian, the Modern Kleinian, and the Independent, to again try to determine whether their clinical work does or does not represent a convergence or common ground of clinical relatedness, as opposed to a divergence into theory-determined different kinds of clinical interventions. To make such comparison and contrast more feasible, each presentation was supposed to be around a single analytic hour in which clearcut oedipal issues were evidenced. For reasons that I make clear in this chapter, I begin with consideration of the Contemporary Freudian analyst, then turn to the Kleinian analyst, and finally the Independent analyst.

## The Freudian Analyst

The Freudian analyst's presentation began with a series of technical-theoretical disclaimers, namely (1) that her clinical approach, though rooted in developmental thinking, gives priority to the analysis of the "here-and-now" with reconstruction of childhood states being used only to provide a temporal dimension to the patient; (2) that the concepts of the infantile neurosis and the transference neurosis have, with nearly all the British colleagues, pretty much fallen by the board; (3) that preoedipal factors inevitably color and are intertwined with oedipal conflicts; (4) that truly neurotic patients are today a rarity in analytic practice; and (5) that triangular situations are not necessarily oedipal in nature, here referring not just to the (triangular) necessity of negotiating a relationship with two others who have an independent relationship with each other but probably also to the French conception of the oedipal situation as representing the negotiation of the issues of "the double difference," the difference in genders and the difference in generations. I list all these statements because, in ensemble, they can represent a convergence in thinking of all three of the main theoretical streams in British psychoanalysis, meaning that they could be stated quite comparably by representatives of both the modern Kleinian and the Independent groups.

Given that, do we then still discern clinical differences in conception and in technique? To some extent we do. The Freudian analyst states that in the search for an hour in which oedipal conflicts can be seen in pure culture, she found an "especially obliging patient" to describe. The patient is a married man with two children, a physician, in treatment for dissatisfactions with his life, tendencies to depression and isolation, and some marital difficulties. In the hour presented he began by expressing concern for the analyst's cold and her "bunged-up" sinuses, to the extent that he made her feel slightly guilty for exposing him to her cold rather than canceling the hour as her husband had urged. He then talked about the new attractive young woman patient waiting to see the analyst's husband (also an analyst) in the shared waiting room, remarking that the analyst's husband appeared less friendly than usual, somewhat disdainful, and possibly annoyed with him, when collecting his own patient in the waiting room. This was followed by comments about the stiffness in his own neck, with the thought that maybe he should see his osteopath for a manipulation, and then finally a dream in which his wife Stephanie appeared particularly sexually attractive and from which he awoke with anxiety. In his associations to the dream, the patient was first struck that Stephanie looked a little different than usual, that she had short hair that reminded him of a photograph of his mother as a young woman. He then recalled a nightmare from childhood when, after seeing a circus, he had dreamt that his bedroom door opened and a large tiger, just like the one that had jumped in the ring at the circus, burst into the room.

The analyst's own parallel associations were to her own new shorter haircut and her conclusion that the patient was suddenly bringing in clearly oedipal material, which had not been much in evidence before, in which a linkage existed among his wife, his mother, and his analyst that aroused excitement and consequent anxiety. The tiger could readily represent the sadistic frightening and punishing response to the patient's arousal. But here the Freudian analyst "decided to wait before offering an interpretation, as I was not sure what had prompted all this material and why it was coming to the surface during this particular session." In this more hesitant and restrained approach to interpretation, in deciding to await further unfolding before intervening, this analyst seemed typically more "Freudian" (ego psychological) than might be characteristic of her colleagues with differing theoretical allegiances.

And the material did unfold further. The patient talked about his partial impotence in attempted love-making the previous night, with consummation achieved only when his wife performed fellatio on him, which she seemed to enjoy; however, he felt guilty, that she would be angry that he had ejaculated, and also embarrassed that he would need to confess this interaction to the analyst. At this point the Freudian analyst in her own mind made further connections between her patient's ejaculating into his wife's mouth, and his comments about his own stiff neck and his analyst's bunged-up sinuses and postnasal drip. However, the analyst again decided to wait before interpreting her patient's unconscious sexual wishes toward her because she wanted to circumvent his tendencies toward a defensive intellectualizing and she wanted to be more sure that she could present her interpretation in an emotionally convincing manner. All she did say at this point was that she felt that in some way the patient had his wife, his mother, and his analyst all mixed up in his mind. This is an expectant and exploratory intervention again much more characteristic of those within the ego psychological paradigm, as technically originally codified by Fenichel, of working slowly from the surface to the depth and making interpretive interventions only at the point where the unconscious material is literally just about at the point of emerging into consciousness.

Again the patient went on, talking about the attractive new woman awaiting his analyst's husband and about the magazine article about beauty contests that he had been reading when the analyst's husband came for his patient. This was where the patient so strongly felt the analyst's husband's disapproval and his own embarrassment—almost as if he had been caught in the act. From this he went on to his childhood embarrassment when he was home from school with a cold, resting in his parents' bed, and his father came in and caught him looking at a brochure advertising brassieres that was very exciting to him and he remembered that he had had an erection. Father had actually seemed not to notice and was indeed quite solicitous of him: this brought to the analyst's mind the pleasure she had felt during the previous hour over the patient's progress in the analysis. At this point she offered a first-step interpretive intervention, calling the patient's attention to his own recent expression of pleasure at his analytic progress and the concomitant work promotion that he had just been offered. She noted that all of this aroused his anxiety, with the specific fear that the analyst's husband would be aware of and resent the fact that the patient was now getting along so well with his (the analyst's husband's) wife.

The interpretation could be seen as but a small and an impressively justified inferential step, which indeed opened the way to much convincing confirmatory material. The patient said that he didn't know about the analyst's husband, but he was certainly concerned about a colleague and work rival over whose head he was being promoted. This colleague was angry and had just very clearly snubbed him and certainly couldn't be trusted because he did carry grudges. And further, although the patient was a very careful driver, he did manage to bash in his car fender when driving out of his driveway just this past weekend, which had never happened before. This did link to his habit of minor accidents when in the throes of guilt feelings, like mislaying keys or forgetting appointments. He should certainly try to make peace with his colleague and rival at work.

Only at this point did the Freudian analyst feel emboldened to widen the interpretive network significantly, adding that perhaps there was a part of the patient that wished to have his analyst's husband out of the way so that he could have her all to himself, which immediately made him feel anxious so that he would feel the wish to make his peace with her husband also. After that the rest fell into place. The patient said laughingly that he would hate to have a hostile husband just around the corner; he associated to a nephew's hernia surgery in the preceding few days, and his anxieties over his own hernia surgery when he was only 5. The surgeon was a friend of his father's, and he himself was very frightened and very concerned to check the wound, which seemed so enormous when they changed the dressing. This was finally then related to the patient's specific castration anxiety and childhood concern for his penis and to the linked fears that the angry husband of his analyst would take revenge for his sexual excitement both with the female patient in the waiting room and with his analyst. All this material was triggered by his promotion and being then more successful than his father had been, about which he was always guilty and around which he always expected retaliation and punishment.

All in all, it was surely a typically oedipal hour with a sequential and stepwise building to interpretive closure, all the while resonating with and adhering closely to the clinical unfolding—and characteristically accomplished within the clinical postulates of what is called in America the ego psychological, and in Britain the Contemporary Freudian, approach. And yet all this was within the framework of the set of technical-theoretical understandings that provided a position statement that could—and would—be equally subscribed to by colleagues from within the Kleinian and the Independent theoretical positions.

## The Kleinian Analyst

I turn next to the Kleinian presentation because if there are differences in approach—and indeed it turns out that there are—they will likely emerge most sharply in this Freudian-Kleinian juxtaposition. To begin with, the oedipal configuration in the Kleinian analyst's material is much less immediately self-evident. Although discernible and emerging with increasing clarity over the course of the hour, it also seems, certainly in the earlier parts of the hour, much more a matter of inference and construction. The patient is a married professional woman with two children, in a seemingly stable marriage, but with very similar complaints to the patient in Freudian analysis: depressed feelings and a sense of purposelessness in life, with, in this case, some psychosomatic or at least bodily manifestations of recurring pains in her arm and shoulder, at times severe enough to keep her home from work. The hour presented comes from the first week after a summer vacation break. The patient couldn't get to the first session of the week because of a failure in child care arrangements that distressed her greatly, and then she arrived late and very distressed to the second session, complaining loudly about the London traffic (she comes from a long way out in the suburbs). In the following sessions of the week the patient spoke about how miserable and disconnected she had been feeling over the long summer break, and for no good reason. She just felt a mess, and incidentally made no mention of the new striped wallpaper with which the consulting room had been redecorated in the summer—an omission that the analyst noted and felt to be very significant.

The last, the Friday, session of the week began with the analyst keeping the patient waiting three minutes at the beginning of the hour. When the patient began by talking of the absolutely horrible traffic that made it difficult to get to her session that day, the analyst said, "I knew she was talking about a real external event, but I felt sure she also was speaking about her response to being kept waiting." To the Freudian analyst that would no doubt have seemed a very large inferential leap. The Kleinian analyst, however, interpreted immediately, saying that she thought her keeping the patient waiting that morning was horrible to her, as if there were also some kind of traffic jam right in this room blocking her access to her analyst. It is this immediate construction and interpretation presented with a sense of real conviction that to those outside its framework can sound typically or stereotypically Kleinian, and the patient herself responded first with a silence. The patient then stated in an irritated voice that she had felt panicky and indeed had wondered whether she had come at the wrong time and would not find her analyst present, but then in a change of voice remarked that it was nonsensical and ridiculous to feel that way (presumably over only a three-minute delay).

This led to the analyst's feeling distanced and put down, perhaps at the lack of wholehearted agreement with the interpretation? The analyst then returned to her interpretive tack, stating that she thought the patient had been trying to convey her feelings but that something inside had interfered and blocked her. This interpretation in turn led the patient to shift to the somatic pain in her arm and shoulder and her more intense desire to get rid of that, if she had to choose which distress to get rid of. This led the analyst to feel "uncomfortably useless," especially since she was unable to do anything about the patient's painful arm and at that point the analyst (perhaps wisely?) drew back and desisted.

The patient then went on to comment on the new wallpaper for the first time, the redecorating of the consulting room during her summer absence, and the similarity to the wallpaper in her childhood home where all her succeeding siblings were born. She remembered the deliberate messing up of that familiar wallpaper by rubbing her spit on it as well as her spilling cod-liver oil all over the sheets of her bed and how angry her mother got, shouting at her. And this led then to her sense of separateness from Mother, for her bedroom was at the other end of a long corridor from the parents' bedroom and in fact jutted out almost into the next-door neighbors' house. At this point the analyst thought, but again refrained from directly interpreting, that the patient was feeling at the far end of a long corridor from her analyst because of the holiday *and* because of being kept waiting—as if the three-minute wait was somehow in the same realm (or even equivalent to?) the whole summerlong separation. All this would make the patient feel lonely with a father and mother off somewhere away and with her only able to mess things up with her finger, and the Kleinian analyst felt that there was a conflation of the parental home, other people's houses, and her analytic home. All this she did not say at that point and the patient went on to the excitement of childhood masturbation and being caught at it by her father who was not excited by her but was instead angry and disgusted.

Here the analyst felt that what was of primary importance at the moment was not the memory of masturbation and sexual excitement, but rather the patient's description of what she did when she felt far away from her parents, which was comparable to what she was thrown into now by the analyst's lateness on top of the summer holiday; this was again a lifting of the lateness into almost a co-equal event in its intrapsychic reverberations. All this together led the analyst to interpret that her own lateness that day had hurt the patient so much, as if someone was keeping her away from her analyst, that she had deflected these hurt feelings into her arm, that it was all too much to handle, especially being aware that someone else had been inside the analyst's room, redecorating it, inside the analyst doing things, while the patient had to wait outside. Again, what I would take to be a considerable inferential leap, couched of course in a clearly Kleinian language of bodily projections and introjections. However, it did seem to resonate with the patient, who quietly agreed, which apparently she did not do so directly very often. This encouraged the analyst to elaborate further, linking the patient's messing up her parents' house as a child to the wish to mess up her analyst's house out of the poignant loneliness and jealousy she felt at being excluded, with the mobilization then of her defensive anger in response to those hurts.

This then led the patient to memories of childhood sexual play with a little girlfriend and their mutual sexual miseducation that left them with the idea that adults needed a tube of some kind to consummate sexual activity and their subsequent search in the cupboard for the proper tube to play "Mummy and Daddy." When the analyst said how terrible to feel like the little girl at the end of the corridor or in the analytic waiting room with the defensive switch of imagining herself to be the Daddy who gets to be with Mummy after all (i.e., the lifting of the interpretation into the clearly oedipal realm), the patient suddenly remembered the previous night's dream. In the dream the patient was with a fellow male student who had once had a crush on her. In the dream they were having an affair, they were in love, she was tremendously happy, and the analyst was somewhere around in the background. The patient had then awakened in the middle of the night, felt very happy, and her arm and shoulder pain were gone, though after she got up to use the toilet, the pains had returned. In association to the dream, the patient remembered that her own original crush on that man had come during the analytic Christmas break and thus directly under the analyst's eyes, i.e., a confirmatory set of clearly oedipal dream associations in response to the analyst's oedipal interpretation. To add to matters, both knew that the man worked at a clinic where the analyst also worked.

This led to the summary interpretations of the hour. The analyst stated that the affair with the fellow student in the dream felt like a love affair with the analyst, i.e., the analyst equated herself with the young man. But this love affair with the analyst was without sexuality or jealousy, without messing up; it was with a student connected with the analyst, and the analyst herself was in the background. The "tube" had been found that enabled patient and the analyst to be sexless but perfect lovers, a relationship was created with the analyst not spoiled by a father, and therefore it was happy and without jealousy, and without pain in her arm as well. The patient made no direct response, but stated, more indirectly, that she was indeed sad, that the analyst was and always would be only her analyst, never her lover, that it was all just a dream that she wanted to hold onto in the night.

At the end of her account of this hour, the analyst added a coda explaining and defending her understanding of the material and her manner of intervention. She thought that her keeping the patient waiting at the start of the session, even if only for three minutes, coming after the long difficult summer break and added to by the consulting room redecoration in her absence, "plunged this patient into an intensely painful inverted oedipal jealousy." She felt the patient to be feeling profoundly distressed, abandoned, and left out at the end of a long corridor, far away from the parents together in intercourse and making babies, i.e., a "straightforward and classically oedipal scenario." And the analyst added then her view, which she of course interpreted to the patient, of the patient's defensive handling of this pain and hurt, the patient's sexual excitement (her masturbation), her identification with the sexual father, and her imagining the blissful nonsexual union with the analyst.

Because of the construction element in the interpretations and its larger inferential leaps, it is less clear in this account than in that of the Freudian analyst how fully the Kleinian analyst has been in empathic attunement with the patient's ongoing psychic states during that hour, and there are momentary disjunctions at which points the analyst did pause and wait. However, overall the analysis clearly seemed to move in the elucidation of what seemed to be the central issue, which was felt by both, of the patient's alienation and difficulty in reconnecting after the long summer break during which the analyst and her husband would be far away doing things together and during which as well other people were inside and "messing up" the consulting room. Whether the three-minute (anxious?) wait at the start of the session added even a triggering impact to all this is an issue that each reader can decide separately. What *is* clear is a real difference in technical approach between the Freudian and Kleinian analysts: the more tentative, careful, slow, and stepwise interpretive progression of the Freudian analysis and the bolder, more certain, and clearly more far-ranging interpretive thrust (the greater inferential leaps) of the Kleinian analysis. That this distinct difference is very much in line with the usual characterization of technical differences between the Freudian or ego psychological approach and the Kleinian approach is clear enough. To what extent this represents a theory-driven difference in technique, readily separating the Freudian from the Kleinian, and, if so, to what extent such a difference plays a decisive role in separating the manner in which Freudian and Kleinian analyses progress, or to what extent this is simply a fortuitous difference in analytic style or temperament between two British colleagues is of course, a crucial question and one to which I return after discussing the presentation of the Independent analyst.

## The Independent Analyst

The Independent Group originally consisted of that large cluster of British analysts who could identify neither with the Freudian nor with the Kleinian position, but who remained independently outside of both, resisting even being designated as a group. They did, however, finally organize as the Middle Group, now renamed the Independent Group, and have been known for their object-relational perspective with a central focus both on the evolving internalized object relationships as the prime organizers of personality formation and on the salience of real events, including the inevitable traumata marking the developmental process, in shaping the way in which these internalized object relationships become established. The Independent analyst began his presentation with a discussion of the trauma of termination of analysis, with its loss and consequent mourning as a major real event in every analysis, made of course more difficult and poignant where such issues had played a significant role in the patient's earlier life history. This kind of concern would expectedly be more to the fore with the members of this group than with a Freudian or Kleinian, although the modern proponents of these other theoretical positions also of course take real-life events and real-life traumata into serious account.

The patient in the Independent analysis, like the others, suffered depression, in this instance, subsequent to a divorce; in her marriage she had had a masochistic posture, dutifully looking after the children and not allowed to work by her very successful husband. She was deeply sad, in a state of chronic mourning except when briefly hypomanic, and also suffered with somatic symptoms. Her whole growing up was restricted and sad, dominated by a chronically ill father who she was told might readily take a turn for the worse if she was naughty or noisy. In keeping with her analyst's object-relational perspective, she was described as always relentlessly in search of the real person behind the analyst's professional mask and resented interpretations which she saw as proof of the analyst's uncaringness—again, a typically Independent group perspective with its lesser focus on the salience of interpretation and a concomitant greater reliance on the properly constructed "holding environment," a concept from Winnicott, one of the major figures in the early coalescing object-relational focus.

The patient was seen to be always in search of a strong man in a position of authority, but would get excited and triumphant if she could then expose his weakness, which would mean that he was only human after all. The perfect analytic stance was a replica of her mask-like and unresponsive father. One of the reasons given for the patient's constant pressure to end the analysis was that the patient could then fantasize a different (real) relationship with the analyst. Yet each time she set a tentative termination date, to which the analyst would agree, she would get deeply depressed; this convinced her that perhaps she would never be able to end, but would have to helplessly come forever. After several repetitions of this scenario, the analyst finally told her that she *should not* terminate, but should remain at least another full year. The patient initially protested this "cruel sentence," but then quickly accepted it with real relief and entered into the most productive year of the analysis. The analyst felt that he had finally—by his action, not interpretation—undercut the patient's tenacious belief that he had never really wanted her as a patient and was always secretly seeking to rid himself of her. In the work of that last year the patient exhibited an intense competitiveness with the analyst, over who would make interpretations first, over showing how smart she was, longing to bring pleasure and pride to her father-analyst. This in turn was linked to her feeling that the coincidence of her birth and the onset of his chronic illness made her responsible for her father's disabled state.

The patient began the reported session, a few months before termination, saying that she had seen a mother at school who, as a youngster, had seen a previous therapist at the Tavistock who had not been at all helpful. From the description the patient had surmised and then confirmed that the previous therapist had been her present analyst, and this made her feel excited and triumphant that she was the better therapist. But she then had to immediately switch to another family she had seen where her analyst had also been the prior therapist and had been very helpful. She hadn't wanted to tell him this at first because he would feel too proud; it all showed how bitchy she really was. Here the analyst directly interpreted that she had a need to create idols, but was excited when they crashed down, just like Father did. The patient in turn elaborated this. She feared in the beginning that the analyst would be weak and that she could teach him, but he turned out to be stronger than she thought and could see through all her tricks and never gave way to emotional displays—in contrast to her previous therapist whom she had once reduced to tears.

This led to a closely interactive sequence with the analyst in which he progressively enlarged his interpretive thrust —that the patient had felt that she could tell him about his useless consultation without fearing that he would be brought to tears; that her search for weakness in men (husband, father, analyst) was a wish not only to triumph but also to find a weak father whom she could look after, replacing Mother— the oedipal motif; and that, in response to the patient's statement that Mother enjoined her to pray for her father nightly because he might die, she probably believed that by her birth or her badness she had caused his illness. To this last the patient replied that, fantasy or not, she had truly caused the illness because without her it would not have happened. The analyst then capped this interpretive sequence by pointing out that today the patient had to make him into the father who was knocked down (the bad consultation) but then also quickly revived him (the good consultation). In all, an interpretive sequence building in much the same fashion as in the Freudian analyst's reported hour and likewise enlarging in close touch with the patient's immediately presenting material.

At this point the patient acknowledged that she was now feeling less sad, that termination need not be thought of in funeral terms, but more like a graduation. She had gone to a funeral the day before, but it was a humanist service of the kind she would like for herself. She did not believe in an afterlife, but did now believe in a psychoanalytic after-life. She had created a paranoid structure around herself to convince herself, via her several premature efforts at termination, that she was being abandoned all over again. She no longer needed that structure; the extra year had indeed given her hope that she need no longer consider herself unloved and unlovable.

By now the main work of the hour had been done. The patient was thinking of graduation day, of how much work they had done, but she was nonetheless still the same person. Actually she was glad of that too. She then spoke of a lifelong nightmare-like feeling of unspecified failure and nameless dread accompanied by massive guilt. That was now greatly faded, and she could enjoy things more. She has taken up swimming again and is glad that she had some lessons from the instructor. This enabled the Independent analyst to add at the end that he had been the instructor, to which the patient rejoined that he had never instructed her, but had just been the water (echoes of Winnicott's "holding environment"?).

The analyst then added his reflections on the state of the analysis. He felt the central transference dynamic to be the quest for potent men whose weaknesses she could then expose. She identified with a morose and sick father and was herself internally dead. She desperately wanted a well father, to make him well while also feeling intensely rivalrous with him. She was always a Poor Little Thing who didn't have a proper Daddy. In this specific session where the patient discovered the analyst's past secret professional life, she had found him bad (impotent) but also good (potent). She could readily acknowledge her jealousy and her wish to be destructively attacking. All this had been repeatedly interpreted over time. This time the analyst focused on the reparative wish to find Father wanting, so that she could then take over Mother's function to care for and rehabilitate him—the oedipal interpretation that clearly seemed to advance the analytic work.

## Concluding Comments

How then to compare this presentation with the Freudian and Kleinian hours? There is clearly discernible the greater explanatory consideration given in this object-relational framework to the impact of the real lifelong traumata experienced centrally by the patient: the father's severe illness across the whole span of the patient's growing-up years, with her own felt responsibility for causing it, regularly reinforced by Mother's cautions that her naughtinesses and noisinesses would worsen the father's condition. There were also the hints in the setting of the context of the hour that interpretations needed to be employed with caution since they could so easily be felt as expressions of coldness and unempathic objectifying and that concern for the caretaking and nurturing relationship (here Winnicott and Balint) should be equally kept in mind. But the actual interpretive style in the moment-to-moment interactions seemed very much like the stepwise progression of the Freudian analysis, which built gradually both to greater depth and fullness. What are thought of as the special hallmarks of the object-relational approach—especially with the sicker and more regressed patients that, as far as I could tell from the limited material presented, this patient certainly was not—the chariness and restraint in interpretation while the regressive potential of the patient would be allowed to unfold within the support- ive and containing therapeutic relationship was simply here not in evidence.

What then is my overview on the juxtaposition of the three sessions? Clearly all three presentations dealt with the interpretive uncovering of the oedipal dynamic, in more clear-cut form in the Freudian hour and more to be extracted and brought into focus in the Kleinian and Independent analyses. All three addressed this oedipal dynamic through the phenomena of conflict and compromise, of impulse and defense, of inner and outer object world, of reality and fan- tasy. The interpretive style of the Freudian and Independent analysts involved a slower and more tentative step-by-step building, closely tied to the associative flow of the psychic material that likewise, in stepwise fashion, emerged in the analytic interaction. The interpretive steps were less infer- ential; they were more immediately evident in the material. The interpretive style of the Kleinian analyst was bolder: more declarative, more far ranging and with greater infer- ential leaps. This led to momentary disjunctions between ana- lyst and patient that, however, seemed in each instance to be recovered from. Each of the three reached comparable points in accomplishing the interpretive aims of the pre- sented hours in relation to the oedipal material elaborated in them.

It is easy enough to call these different interpretive styles typically—or again, stereotypically—Freudian or Kleinian, but there is nothing inherent in ego psychological or in Kleinian theory that requires these differences in approach; that is, they are not theory-driven or theory-determined. They could as well be differences in personal style and temperament, and it is equally plausible that the same distinction in interpretive style (as between the Freudian and Kleinian analysts, for example) could be found between two representatives of the Contemporary Freudian group or between two of the Modern Kleinian group. At least this has been my own experience, over many years, of listening to and studying clinical presentations by representatives of all these groups, over the whole range of training and experience, and in all of the regions of the world. Certainly, it is also clear that the real *theoretical* differences among the ego psychological (Contemporary Freudian), object-relational (Independent), and Modern Kleinian metapsychologies are not evident in the actual descriptions of the *clinical* interactions in the three consulting rooms presented to us, nor have these different metapsychologies been coercive in framing the interpretive direction of the three presenting analysts, though each of course has inevitably been operating within the guiding framework of an espoused theoretical perspective that can at times be discerned in the choice of interpretive language. All of which still leaves this debate over how tightly theory determines technique of course unresolved.

I need to end then with the same kind of caveat I expressed in the final section of my Rome address. Of course, individual differences of style, temperament, and how the essentials of tact and timing, and of choice and selection are experienced and expressed are present and visible in these three representative British analysts. That is, after all, part of our common-sense knowledge of the bewildering diversity and range of human nature and of specifically psychoanalytic experience. And of course, though here far less obviously, some theory-linked differences in choice of interventions and in the style and language of interventions also do exist and can often enough be discerned and identified.

My contention is not that no such differences exist. Rather, it is that the overarching commonality of our clinical approach to the phenomena of the analytic interaction in the consulting room transcends both our individual differences of style and temperament as unique people and the conceptual differences of our theoretical explanatory frameworks and brings us together as identifiably all psychoanalysts doing the common work of psychoanalysis in comparable enough ways. I wish that this particular comparative clinical exercise had brought us further toward consensus on this conviction that I hold than the old Scottish verdict—not (yet) proven.

### References

Wallerstein, R. S. (1988). One psychoanalysis or many? *International Journal of Psycho-Analysis* 69:5–21.
—— (1990). Psychoanalysis: the common ground. *International Journal of Psycho-Analysis* 71:3–20.

# IV

## COMMENTARY:
## BRITISH ANALYSTS

# 9

## Commentary by
## Marion Burgner

### Introduction

I am rather uneasy about being described in this book as a Contemporary Freudian rather than simply as an analyst of the British Society. Certainly my training in both child and adult analysis was within that group, and I am temperamentally attuned and sympathetic to many of its theoretical models and postulates, though by no means all of them. But I am able to use, critically and elastically, conceptual models claimed to originate from the other two groups when such models facilitate my and the patients' understanding of their individual psychic predicaments. In addition, there is considerable variation and discrepancy in approach between members of any one group in the Society.

It is important for me, as a practicing child and adult analyst, to know that I have a substantial and accessible body of theory. But it has always seemed of equal importance that I should be capable of an analytic stance in the consulting room that does not lean too heavily and too automatically upon any one analytic formulation. In such a desirable analytic mental set, John Keats's (1817) definition of "negative capability" is relevant: "that is when a man is capable of being in uncertainties, mysteries, doubts, without any irritable reaching after fact and reason" (p. 72). My endeavor not to be too dependent on or attached to any one theory is, in part, connected with an awareness that the theories we are taught, the theories we gradually become most attracted to, the theories that inform our understanding of our daily clinical work, practically all of these are in essence conceptual models of the mind, metaphors that, as Wallerstein (1988) writes, have been created "in order to satisfy our variously conditioned needs for closure and coherence and overall theoretical understanding" (p. 15).

It is nonetheless facilitating to have, for instance, a structural theory in order to understand in the mind of any one person the compelling pressures and wishes, the rational and adaptive capacities, and the guilty and painful responses; but even in such a simplistic view of the tripartite structural division of the mind, it is clear that I have departed from Freud's original view of the id as the instinctual axis of the mind, the structure that is the prime reservoir of psychic energy. And this sort of departure does inform one's working approach. We have to be careful not to discard theories simply because we tire of them and need something innovative, but we have to be flexible enough both in our thinking and in our analytic work to use conceptual models, both the old and the new, only if they are viable clinically and theoretically.

Moreover, clinical work has to avoid the obvious pitfall of simply replicating theory. There inevitably exists a mental backdrop of theoretical formulations, but ideally, these have to be held at a preconscious level while following the thrust, frequently confused and confusing, of the patient's material. Essentially, theorizing comes later, perhaps not even quite clearly when I think afterward about an analytic session, but much more explicitly when I need to formulate in writing or to present it in discussion with colleagues.

Sandler (1983) aptly stresses the multiple dimensions of meaning of psychoanalytic concepts, and he suggests that such elasticity does much to hold divergent psychoanalytic theory together, enabling it to tolerate and absorb theoretical changes. He writes too about the incomplete nature of psychoanalytic theory in that it has to encompass and explain more than its relevance to the clinical and pathological modes: "To try to satisfy all 'explanatory intents' with one comprehensive theory is clearly impossible, and I would urge the view that we have a body of ideas, rather than a consistent whole, that constitutes psychoanalytic theory." He emphasizes the centrality of the work we have to do "within the whole compass of psychoanalytic thinking," that such work means for most of us that "the theory needs to be a clinically, psychopathologically, and technically oriented one which also includes a central preoccupation, not only with the abnormal, but with the normal as well" (p. 37).

Sandler undoubtedly addresses something fundamental that may lie behind the plan for this book—that three analysts from different groups within the British Society would inevitably use psychoanalytic concepts differently in their clinical work. Yet, the divergence and, for that matter, the convergence of conceptualization in the three presented cases are seen more in technique than in conceptualization. Conceptualization may certainly be seen to be of some consequence in all three presentations, but there is a palpable difference in approach between the Kleinian and Freudian analyst in terms of timing of interpretations and the amount said to their patients. I would like to learn from both analysts the exact time that elapsed between the beginning of the session and when they each spoke first and what their rationale was for this intervention. The Kleinian analyst seemed to take only a moment or so to speak, whereas for the Freudian analyst there is a long time gap. Although she is actively making associative links in her own thinking, she begins to speak at a point well into the session, possibly at the halfway point or more, and it is a facilitating rather than an interpretive comment; it is after several more communi-

cations from the patient that she actually begins to pull together the patient's material in a coherent interpretation. The
work of the Independent analyst seems different again in
terms of technique, as he apparently intervened regularly in
response to what the patient said. Another technical difference is that the Freudian analyst seems more preoccupied
than the other two analysts with the multifaceted psychic
conflict in her patient's mind and the central oedipal conflict between being a professionally and sexually successful
man and being punished and diminished for such achieve-
ments; this conflict is addressed both in the transference and
reconstructively by analyst and patient.

It is important to differentiate carefully between theoretical models and developmental criteria such as phases of
development. Such phases, though weighted with observa-
tional and descriptive rather than explanatory data, are in-
valuable in broad terms for assessment of the child's and then
the adult's developmental progress. We are all aware of the
vital organizational value of the oedipal experience in the
structuring of internal object relationships. One of my interests in understanding development—from infancy, early and
later childhood, through the vicissitudes of adolescence
to adulthood—has been the fate of the Oedipus complex
(Burgner 1985). Indeed, I would no longer label it a complex in the classical sense, but rather *a distorted or pseudo-
oedipal* mental configuration, and the dyadic emphasis between child and mother remains of paramount importance.
This distorted emphasis is carried forward in development
so that ensuing phases also have a pseudo quality about them;
there may be triadic interaction at the time when we first
expect oedipal emergence, but such interaction remains at
the level of triangulation and does not ripen into a full-bodied
oedipal relationship. It is this persistence of structures and
modes of behavior from earlier phases, with a corresponding lack of dominance of oedipal relationships, that we quite

frequently encounter in our child and adult patients. Many of these patients have experienced relative failures in the first three years of life within the mother–child relationship, in the sense of the mother's capacities and predictable responsiveness, her reflexive understanding of the child's mental states, and in the child's gradual internalization of the containing parental objects. Subsequent psychic development is skewed, and one of the important factors in the ensuing impeded separateness from the internal primary object is an emphasis on dyadic rather than triadic internal relationships.

With such issues in mind, I consider the three presentations in turn.

### The Presentation of the Independent Analyst

The Independent analyst sets his oedipal session within the wider context of the termination of an analysis. I disagree with his assertion of a lack of useful papers on termination. Rather, there is now, following Freud's (1937) seminal paper, "Analysis Terminable and Interminable," an abundance of interesting and useful papers on issues concerning termination written from clinical, theoretical, and technical viewpoints. I assume, though he does not specifically state this, that the analyst, in giving his clinical session this particular emphasis, implicitly believed that every developmental move carries something of an inherent ending within it. In addition, his patient, Mrs. T., a woman in her forties, in her repeated postponement of termination of the analysis was unable to face the real oedipal and preoedipal deprivations as well as the loss of the analyst in the transference, the analyst to whom she relates as both Mother and Father. In the particular circumstances of Mrs. T.'s life, the father's restricting, perhaps paralyzing, illness loomed large and terrifying,

firstly in the pregnant mother's mind and then overwhelm-
ingly as a physical and increasingly mental presence in the
patient's own experience of him. It is then also to be understood that as an infant and a child she did not experience
herself, nor was she experienced, as a priority for the mother,
who had invariably to be watchful of the incapacitated father.
I can well understand that the Independent analyst's decision, following Michael Balint, to give this woman another
complete year of analysis after her several abortive attempts
to terminate was of marked importance in enabling the
analyst–patient couple to have "the most productive year of
the entire analysis."

In the session under discussion, Mrs. T. finally accepted
that her marriage was at an end, a marriage that had in reality ended thirteen years before. Although this statement has
initially to be considered within the context of the analytic
ending in some months time, it could also be viewed as an
acceptance (and all such acceptances are by their very nature
relative) of the more painful and corroding aspects of
the original failures in her oedipal and, more important,
preoedipal experience. She could not in reality make good
her "reparative wish in taking over Mother's function in caring for and rehabilitating Father," nor could she continue
to endlessly try and actualize this wish within the analysis.
But she could perhaps allow herself to experience analytic
care and rehabilitation in relation both to her body and her
mind and thus be enabled to leave the analysis less self-
damaged and less damaging to others.

The analytic session is one in which Mrs. T. first dimin-
ishes and then reinstates the analyst as an effective and potent male, an approach that the Independent analyst views
as commensurate with the father transference; he takes it into
an oedipal constellation by interpreting that her fantasy is
of replacing the mother so that she is in the superior position of being able to take care of the damaged father. How-

ever, it is also possible to consider this segment of analytic material in terms of her regret and anger that this same damaged, yet loved, father has always been too weak and ineffectual to protect her from and compensate for the uncaring mother. Thus, the analyst in the transference could as much represent the rejecting mother who is then experienced in wish-fulfilling fantasy as loving and helpful. Certainly both aspects of the oedipal fantasy have to be interpreted, since this is invariably an aspect of the normal oedipal struggle, let alone of the flawed oedipal constellation in this woman—the parent who in fantasy has to be disposed of is in reality also a loved parent of identificatory and affective value. For Mrs. T. a further complication is that the mother whom she wishes to be rid of is the less damaged and vulnerable of the two parents; to be left with the frighteningly diminished father would be too much to bear for the 3- to 4-year-old child within the 40+-year-old adult woman.

My difficulty with this clinical presentation is that I remain uncertain whether it is an oedipal session as such. My uncertainty is not predicated on the Independent analyst being from a different group, but rather on my reading the material from an alternative clinical and theoretical viewpoint: that essentially Mrs. T.'s dilemma, which has perhaps informed her life, is contained in her search for the strong father who would stand protectively between the mother and herself. This is a preoedipal issue that obstructs oedipal development.

### The Presentation of the Kleinian Analyst

In reading this careful and detailed presentation of a woman patient, I feel I am in the consulting room participating in a dense and meaningful psychoanalytic exchange.

In this session held at the end of a first week after the long summer break, the patient, Mrs. D., felt "panicky" while waiting three minutes into the session, "in a mess, bad," but condemns herself for these feelings. The pain in her arm and shoulder comes to her notice. The analyst feels "uncomfortably useless" at being unable to "cure" the pain, but it could well be that the patient, aware of the analyst's uselessness for her—the absence, lateness and, as it turns out much more fundamentally, her experienced betrayal—has transmuted her pain from an unbearable psychic mental state into a physical pain that could be effectively treated by someone other than the analyst; her awareness of this internal situation is then affectively conveyed to the analyst.

The patient makes her first reference to the new wallpaper and recalls similar paper in a house she lived in as a child; it was in a bedroom she shared with a younger brother. Next she recalls the messes she made and the layout of the family house. The Kleinian analyst perceptively interprets the distance the patient experiences in her mind between herself as a little girl and the parental couple (the analyst and the partner assigned to her). In the implicit, and then explicit, reference to masturbation, the analyst considers there is "a kind of masturbation going on right then and there" in the session in which the patient is hoping to excite the analyst. I remain unconvinced of this understanding but, in any event, the analyst thinks it more important that the patient used masturbation as a comfort when she felt far away—from her parents at the other end of the corridor and from her analyst and partner during the summer holiday. Here I question what it is in the patient's actual material that substantiates the analyst's assumption of contemporary masturbation? What I would elaborate on in this interpretation, though at this point probably only in my thinking, is the connection between the allusion to masturbation and the shared room with the brother; there could well have been sexual activity between them too as a rival sexual couple to the parents.

The Kleinian analyst then addresses her three-minute lateness for that session in terms of the patient painfully experiencing the analyst as being with someone else "inside of me, occupying me and doing things with and to me while she had to wait." This could be mostly correct, although I would at this point have given as much emphasis to the trans-mutation of the pain from the psyche to the body, since Mrs. D. seems to be a woman who feels impelled to somatize her unbearable painful feelings and, in this instance at any rate, experiences the pain in her arm and shoulder as very debilitating. I wonder whether it is also a pain connected with guilt over masturbation, over mess and spillage, and even over wishing to strike the analyst dead for the preoedipal and oedipal betrayals she has inflicted on her—after all, Mrs. D. is the oldest of five siblings. Thus, I am stressing the patient's psychic pain, whereas the analyst is talking much more con-cretely about the patient's sexual fantasies in the transference that she, the analyst, understands to be an eroticized one. Again, I am not sure whether this difference is necessarily a group difference as such, but rather more a technical and personal one connected with what aspect of the material one would concentrate on at any particular moment in the analy-sis. And, of course, the Kleinian analyst may rightly respond that she knows her patient and where she was psychically centered at that moment in the session.

The analyst then—correctly—addresses the patient's re-versal of the origin and of the analytic experience; now she is not being messed up, but she makes herself the messer-up-in-chief. Yet, Mrs. D. is a woman who, as a child and in company with all other small children, undoubtedly had proliferating fantasies of what the parents did sexually to-gether, the messes they made together, and their probable harmful attacks on each other. So, although I agree that the patient is at this point in the session experiencing feelings of loneliness, jealousy, and unimportance, she is also now struggling with half-recalled childhood fantasies, which also need to be addressed reconstructively. And here there is a group difference in that I would stress the eventual importance of constructive and reconstructive work in addition to the meticulous analytic work in the here-and-now of the transference.

In fact Mrs. D. goes on to talk about her own sexual activities as a small girl—not overtly with the brother at this point as I surmised above—but with another girl. She describes a tube she used in their play of Mummies and Daddies; however, now she knows she had not understood anything at all. Perhaps she even knew then as she struggled with the wishful phallic fantasy, but she certainly knows now with a painful narcissistic certainty that her negative oedipal overture to Mother is doomed to failure. It is here therefore that I part company with the analyst since the patient is not simply talking about "switching things around in her mind," imagining herself in projective identificatory terms to be the father with the mother. It seems more complicated than that: she claims she was unable to understand anything either about how her mother conceived the babies that kept growing inside her. She relates the dream about the asexual affair with the fellow student, and she is aware of tremendous happiness and the absence of physical pain in her arm and shoulder. But when she goes to the lavatory and becomes aware of the reality of her own female genitals, the pain returns. Although the analyst understands this sequence as consonant with a nonsexual, nonmessy, nonjealous love affair with herself and links it with the small girl's invention of the tube enabling her to be close to her mother, this interpretation fails to address the pain the child feels; and it is not only the "pain of jealousy [in] her mind," but as much the pain resulting from the failure of omnipotence. She cannot understand how to engage with Mother in a phallic way (a negative oedipal constellation), nor does she yet know in positive oedipal terms how to present herself to Father as his desirable sexual partner. So she takes defensive refuge in an asexual and beautiful dream about the male student, a dream in which she also enjoys the presence of the benign, similarly asexual analyst. Perhaps this preoedipal and oedipal material could be addressed both transferentially and historically.

Although Mrs. D. has apparently solved her problem of her messy anger and destructiveness toward the analyst/ mother who leaves her over the holiday and remains so busy that she keeps her waiting, we learn in the next, and last, sequence that there has not been a real solution. Her next association is to the oldest girl next door, from the house she sometimes in fantasy lived in, swinging her around by the arm and wrenching her shoulder out. My question is then: Whom does the girl next door represent? I would suggest that she is both the analyst and the mother whom she has experienced as causing her so much psychic and physical pain.

It is clear that this patient is well engaged with her analyst in this session in struggling with possible solutions to her oedipal dilemma and its preoedipal determinants, a dilemma that is very alive in the transference. I would like, however, to put an important question to the Kleinian analyst: Has she condensed in her work with this patient the two views on the oedipal constellation that I have often heard Kleinian analysts express? As I understand these views, there is an initial oedipal relationship in the second half of the first year between the baby and his or her two parents and then a second oedipal relationship, coinciding in its timing with the Freudian developmental view. And it seems possible, reading her clinical material, that the Kleinian analyst's view of the oedipal experience moves between that of the infant and the child with insufficient discrimination between the two.

In fact, triangulation, which occurs as soon as the infant can affectively, or perhaps perceptually, discriminate between Mother and Father, should not be conflated with the later experience of the oedipal relationship proper.

### The Presentation of the Freudian Analyst

With this presentation, I am of course—despite my various disclaimers at the beginning of this chapter—on more familiar ground and I fully share her stated views. First, although rooted in a developmental perspective, we still have whenever possible to concentrate our work on what is happening between patient and analyst in the consulting room during that specific session. Second, the so-called infantile neurosis, the classical oedipal complex, is not viable on its own, neither conceptually nor affectively, as central to the patient's present disturbance. Third, the concept of a coherent transference neurosis has little validity in our work, and it is more appropriate to speak of strong and varied transference feelings. Fourth, rarely, if at all, do we encounter an oedipal conflict in its pure culture since the very nature of the developmental approach rules this out; there are always pre- and postoedipal pressures on the oedipal experience. And fifth, triangulation as such should not be confused with the real oedipal configuration with its relatively sophisticated and conflictual interweaving of relationships and fantasies; triangulation is discernible from early in the infant's life, but it is not fashioned from oedipal fantasies of patricide or matricide with ensuing and conflictual anxieties and guilt.

The Freudian analyst presents a session that is undoubtedly oedipal in its main characteristics. It is also a session in which we are gradually made aware of the virtues of biding one's time, of not leaping in with interim interpretive comments that would have adversely affected the flow of the session. An undoubted aid to this analytic flow was the analyst's recall of her warm feelings toward the patient, Dr. A., at the end of the previous Friday's session and of a feeling of being pleased—presumably both with him and with herself—at the favorable progress of the analytic work. Such feelings are usually silently conveyed to or certainly picked up by the patient without a verbal exchange. Perhaps, however, Dr. A. felt not only gratified but also guilty at his analyst's special regard for him; at any rate, he complained of a stiff neck (linked biblically with hubris), he smashed in the wing of his car, and he failed to maintain an erection with his wife, ejaculating instead in her mouth, an event that seemingly caused him to feel ashamed and fearful of her anticipated anger. And all of this was compounded just before his session by seeing the analyst's husband enter the waiting room to collect his attractive woman patient and casting him, as he experienced it, a disdainful and distanced glance. So, the analyst/mother is experienced as liking him too much while the analyst's husband/father is viewed as capable of anger with the usurper (the patient) and of betrayal of his wife/analyst with his attractive woman patient.

After talking about this encounter in the waiting room, the patient recalls a dream in which his wife looked beautiful and seductive, though he felt anxious on waking since she looked different. He then remembers a nightmare from the age of 12 after seeing a circus performance with his parents, a nightmare in which a large tiger bursts into his bedroom; this image has often haunted him subsequently. The analyst, still silent, wonders to herself whether the tiger represents "some sadistic and frightening aspect of his self." But it seems very possible that, if one understands the thrust of the material as oedipal, the tiger could well represent the powerful avenging father/analyst's husband more than being an aspect of the self. The analyst's husband, the patient then reveals, is also experienced as catching him in flagrante delicto in the waiting room looking at a magazine article about beauty contests, just as his father had caught him, when ill in the parental bed, excitedly looking with an erection at a magazine advertisement for brassieres. This material then is also about his fantasies about the parental couple.

Dr. A. goes on to talk about his fear of his father as a child and of being spoiled by his mother. The analyst then feels convincingly enabled by her recollected countertransference feelings of the previous session to begin her oedipal interpretation, first in connection with the patient's gratitude toward her for their successful work together and hence his ensuing anxiety about her husband's resentment and jealousy. The patient responds by talking about how anxious and guilty he feels toward a colleague who was angry at being passed over for promotion while he, Dr. A., got the job. The analyst returns to her view that it is her husband not the colleague who is central to this particular scenario and that it is her husband whom Dr. A. wishes to have out of the way. Dr. A. continues, as the session comes to an end, to talk about his 5-year-old nephew's hernia operation and to recall his own operation at the same age as well as his fascination with the "enormous wound." The analyst concludes the session by making a comprehensive interpretation of the patient's fear of emasculation, originally by his father and now at her husband's hands. She sees his present anxieties as precipitated by his promotion (in reality he has professionally surpassed his father as well as his colleague), his guilt at their shared and successful analytic work, and his fear of retaliation originally from his father and now from her husband. These feelings are linked to his wishes to steal first the mother and now the analyst and the attractive woman patient.

I have these concerns about the Freudian presentation.

I wonder why the analyst waited quite so long to make her first interpretation and whether her silence could have attenuated the affective strength of the transference. My next comment is about a possible lack of affective delineation, a too careful and measured phrasing in one of her interpretations. I appreciate that this is her individual style, but I would have given more emphasis to the interpretation she makes after the patient describes damaging his car and links this incident with his guilt about being promoted over a colleague's head. Dr. A. has already talked of experiencing the analyst's husband's disdain in the waiting room, the nightmare of the threatening tiger, and his temporary impotence with his wife (linked I surmise, though not explicitly in the session, with his transference fantasies). The analyst then says, "Perhaps there is a part of you that would like to have my husband out of the way so that you can have me all to yourself. But I think this makes you uneasy, and so you feel the need to make your peace with him [her husband] too." Given the strength of Dr. A.'s projections in regard to the husband, I would have aimed for an interpretation that would have conveyed more convincingly and comprehensively the analyst's appreciation of her patient's intensity of feeling—his positive feelings, his guilt, and also his terror of the killing tiger.

My third comment is directed toward the preoedipal tenor of the material. Of course, one can only deal with so much in any one session, but the unusual event of the patient being unable to maintain an erection and then ejaculating in his wife's mouth seems to have something quite new about it for Dr. A. and could well be addressed. Dr. A. is expressing in this, for him, shaming and regressive gesture a contempt for his wife and his analyst as well as a fear of their potency and danger in relation to him. Indeed, the tiger of his 12-year-old nightmare could well represent the oversolicitous engulfing mother and the strict father.

## Concluding Comments

In these three clinical presentations there are certainly aspects of what Wallerstein (1988) calls the "pluralism in theoretical perspectives." There are specific diversities in technique in relation to the timing and frequency of interpretation and in the maintenance of a transferential emphasis as opposed to the additional and judicious use of construction and reconstruction in bringing an eventual coherence to transference interpretations.

These comments are not intended in any way to be supervisory, but only additions or questions or sometimes disagreements with the work presented; and such disagreements are often about technique though occasionally also about theoretical concepts and the validity of their application to the clinical material. I continue the dialectic within the British Psycho-Analytical Society, but since it is offered in the spirit of the 1990s rather than of the historical 1940s when the Controversial Discussions took place (see King and Steiner 1991), I hope it will be accepted accordingly.

## References

Burgner, M. (1985). The oedipal experience: effects on development of an absent father. *International Journal of Psycho-Analysis* 66(3).

Freud, S. (1937). Analysis terminable and interminable. In *Collected Papers*, vol. 5, pp. 316–357. New York: Basic Books, 1959.

Keats, J. (1948). Letter to George and Thomas Keats. In *The Letters of John Keats*, ed. M. B. Forman. London: Oxford University Press.

King, P., and Steiner, R. (1991). *The Freud-Klein Controversies 1941–45*. London: Routledge.

Sandler, J. (1983). Reflections on some relations between psychoanalytic concepts and psychoanalytic practice. *International Journal of Psycho-Analysis* 64(1):37.

Wallerstein R. S. (1988). One psychoanalysis or many? *International Journal of Psycho-Analysis* 69(1):15.

# 10

## Commentary by Michael Parsons

Three leading analysts, one from each group of the famously diverse but somehow cohesive British Society, willing to show themselves at work for us to observe them individually and to compare them with each other—a rich feast! But, as with all exciting menus, we must read carefully if we are to get the most out of what we are offered.

The three groups in the British Society are no more homogeneous than the Society as a whole; and to think that these three individuals represent group viewpoints, so that by reading them we are discovering the theoretical position of, say, the Klein group as a whole, or the technical approach shared by all Independents, would be misleading. The same applies, of course, to the contributions, including this one, of the discussants from the three groups. There are differences within, and overlaps between all three of the Contemporary Freudian, Kleinian, and Independent Groups.

There are also differences between the presentations that may affect our comparison of them. The presentation of the Independent analyst is linked to a particular theoretical concern, that of termination, in addition to the designated oedipal focus. Furthermore the oedipal situation in this case was grossly abnormal, being skewed by the father's severe chronic illness. We are not told of any comparable distortions in the other two cases. The patients are of similar ages (mid-thirties, "fortyish") and are all professional people; but whereas the Freudian and Kleinian analysts' cases had been in their analyses for three years and were continuing, that of the Independent analyst was approaching the end—and a problematic end, at that—of what seems to have been about six years of analysis. So we must be careful about generalizing from these clinical accounts. But there is no denying their richness and there is plenty in them for us to observe, compare, and learn from.

Analysts have one eye on the patient's past history and one on the present-time interaction with the analyst and are always concerned with how to relate them to each other. The Independent analyst's patient begins her session with a long, excited account of seeing, in her professional capacity, a woman who had previously seen the analyst himself. She tried to find out about the consultation with him, experiencing a mixture of superiority and grievance as she did so. She then says that a month previously she had seen another family who had seen him; it seems that she has withheld this information until now. She interprets her own envy and comments on her bitchiness. All this seems very provocative and intrusive. It is striking that, in his response to the patient, the analyst makes no reference to the *quality* of her communication. What was she doing with the analyst in her mind when she ferreted out his old consultations? What is she doing with him in the session as she regales him with the story? These questions are not touched on. Instead the analyst links her idealization and denigration directly to feelings about her father's illness in the past.

The Independent analyst explains that the theme of triumphing over the analyst and then restoring him was extremely familiar. We are nearing the end of several years of analysis, and the analyst writes that such enactments within the session had often been taken up already. It is striking, nonetheless, to compare this with the beginning of the session described by the Kleinian analyst. The patient starts by talking about the traffic and how difficult it is to get to the session. The analyst recognizes that this is a real difficulty, and we know that the patient spends three hours each day traveling to and from her analysis. But the analyst takes it up directly as a reference to the blocked communication in the session. Then there is a noticeable change in the patient's tone of voice. The analyst felt criticized and distanced from the patient, and it is on this sense of what the patient is doing to her that she bases her next intervention. The attention of both analysts may be evenly suspended, but not from the same vertex.

This is not to say, however, that the Kleinian analyst does not deal with history or the Independent analyst with the present-time analytic relationship. The Kleinian analyst's patient moves on to detailed, intimate recollections from her childhood, whereas the patient of the Independent analyst is soon talking about her impression of him and her emotional responses to him. All analytic work must move freely between fact and fantasy, past and present, the transference and other relationships, and here we see just that. But with different analysts that freedom of movement can occur in different ways. The Kleinian analyst refers to the patient's memories "into which she had been plunged by the situation between us." For the Independent analyst, by contrast, it is the patient's historical memories of her father's falling and her head-banging that lead into her feelings about the analytic situation.

Linked to this is a subtle difference about what one actually means by a memory. The Kleinian analyst goes on from the words quoted above to elaborate the "memories" in question: "she was talking about where she is in her mind when she feels I am at the far end of a long corridor from her—because of the holidays, because of keeping her waiting." The patient had described the corridor between her and her parents' bedrooms. That is a childhood memory, but the corridor in her mind is a fantasy. The analyst continues: "I felt aware that in the consulting room there was a little girl and that somewhere in her mind there is a mother and father together. . . . I felt these were important memories."

We see how from this perspective the concept of a memory and that of a fantasy slide in and out of each other and at times seem not to be distinguished, whereas for the Independent analyst the demarcation between them is more definite.

The Freudian analyst begins her presentation with some theoretical remarks about the relation between the present-time analytic experience within the session and the patient's history. She writes that her technical approach "although rooted in developmental thinking, gives priority to the analysis of the 'here and now,' with reconstruction in terms of the specific patient's development being used to provide a temporal dimension to the patient's insight."

All three analysts thus have their own distinctive attitudes to analyzing the here and now and the developmental history, and their own particular ways of moving between them and allowing one to illuminate the other.

The Freudian analyst also states that British analysts do not, in general, use the concept of the transference neurosis in the sense of a replication with the analyst of a specific, focal neurotic pattern from the past. Instead, transference manifestations are considered in a more continuous, general sort of way. I agree. The closest we come to anything like a transference neurosis in these three presentations is perhaps in the Independent session and its analysis of the repetition with the analyst of his patient's distorted relationship to her father. This was certainly central to her pathology, and its repetition in the transference was central to the analysis. Even so, the Independent analyst does not give it a unique, privileged position at the core of the analysis; equally important, for example, is the transference relationship to the rejecting, abandoning mother who might be provoked into ending the analysis.

A passing remark of the Freudian analyst shows us another theoretical shift. She says that in this session her patient was bringing oedipal material "which had not been much in evidence in the analysis before." And this is three years into an analysis conducted by a leading Contemporary Freudian, of all the groups in the British Society the most "classical" in its origins! We are liable to assume that oedipal pathology is nearer the surface, developmentally more evolved, and neurotic rather than psychotic compared to preoedipal pathology, which is deeper, more disturbed, closer to psychotic processes, and developmentally more archaic. However true theoretically, for clinical purposes this division may be misleadingly schematic and oversimplified. The Freudian analyst states emphatically that oedipal conflicts cannot be considered apart from preoedipal factors, and there could be a lively debate about what actually counts as oedipal material. What does the idea of an "oedipal" session, with the implication of some different kind of session that would be "preoedipal," really mean?

The Kleinian analyst's closing reflections on the session she presents recall the comments of the Freudian analyst. The Kleinian analyst writes that material that seemed at first to be straightforwardly and classically oedipal turned out to have preoedipal aspects as well. The patient's anger at being excluded by the parental couple leads directly to regressive material about messing up the walls and dirtying the bed, related to the pregenital use of body products. The patient also seeks a particular kind of intimacy with the analyst: not a sexualized one with a sense of triumph over a rival, but a nonsexual, two-person-only, clearly preoedipal relationship.

With the patient of the Independent analyst, the special features of her father's severe illness and the ending of the analysis complicate the issue. But the case still illustrates how the oedipal and the preoedipal cannot be separated. Her oedipal desire swings between the wish to replace the mother in looking after the ill father and the wish to find a healthy, potent father with whom to develop a more normal relationship. Both wishes, however, involve her in manic reparation to the rejecting mother whom she is terrified will abandon her; abandon her, that is, as a helpless infant who cannot survive on her own. When the patient seeks a relationship in the transference with the father, whether ill or healthy, knocked down or restored, the analyst is bound to appear also as the hating mother, trying to get rid of the daughter not only as an oedipal rival but also as the newborn infant who caused the father's illness, with whom a preoedipal relationship is as intolerable as the oedipal rivalry.

All three presentations thus confirm that oedipal and preoedipal aspects of psychopathology are indissoluble and that any clinical material is bound to contain an expression of both. We must not expect to analyze one separately from the other. How, then, to avoid chaos as we are confronted with a complexity that needs disentangling, but must not be falsely simplified? Members of all three groups in the British Society seem to agree about the problem, these presentations show us different clinical strategies for approaching it. The presentations of the Freudian and Kleinian analysts, coming from similar stages of the analyses of comparable patients, allow us to examine these strategies in some detail.

The Freudian analyst writes that for three years not much oedipal material had appeared in the analysis, and she does not seem to be worried about that. This tells us something about the tempo of the analysis. We have a sense of spaciousness, of something that evolves at its own unhurried rhythm. It is interesting to observe this sense on the smaller scale of the single session. Dr. A. talks about the analyst's cold, about the woman patient in the waiting room, and about whether the analyst's husband was annoyed with him. Then a pause, and he talks about his stiff neck that may need manipulation. Another pause. There is plenty to take up in all this, but the analyst says nothing. The patient goes on to a dream, associates to it about his wife's hair, mentions his mother, and recalls a childhood nightmare. By this stage the analyst tells us that she has a lot of thoughts about the material; but even now she does not intervene: "I decided to wait before offering an interpretation, as I was not sure what had prompted all this material and why it was coming to the surface in this particular session."

Contrast this with the tempo at the beginning of the Kleinian analyst's session. The patient starts by talking about the traffic congestion and how long it took her to get there. The analyst responds by interpreting the patient's feelings about being kept waiting and the blocked communication with the analyst. The patient talks about her feeling of being in a mess, but then pulls herself up. The analyst speaks about what has happened to interfere with what she was saying.

This is a much more interventionist style of analysis, and the rhythm of the analyst's responsiveness is quite different from the Freudian's. The advantages and disadvantages of these ways of analyzing are often discussed, and certain familiar arguments are put forward regularly. Those closer to the viewpoint of the Freudian analyst want the analyst not to be overcertain, not to tell patients what is in their minds, to wait for the nuances of the patients' state of mind to declare themselves, not to be in a hurry to understand. The concept of "negative capability" is bound to get mentioned. Those closer to the style of the Kleinian analyst may say that patients can only face their conflicts if we take up directly the anxiety that stops them from doing so, that the patient needs to see that the analyst is not afraid of the patient's feelings, and that what frightens the patient most and which she cannot confront without help is what most needs bringing into the open, so that we should not wait too long before intervening.

The balance between such arguments is a matter for continual discussion. But comparing these process notes suggests that these different approaches also represent different responses to the complexity of psychoanalytic material, exemplified here by the intertwining of the oedipal and preoedipal. We are faced with the need to comprehend something whose complexity has to be both mastered and respected. I use the word "comprehend" deliberately for its double meaning of to understand and to grasp. We may prefer to watch and wait to understand, while an evolving process gradually allows clarity to appear so that the complexity becomes interpretable. Alternatively we may think that the elements making up the complexity have to be grasped and examined actively before any interpreting can be done.

The Freudian and Kleinian analyst both move between the patient's historical memories and the here and now, the work of both is centered in the transference, and they both interpret oedipal material. Why then do the sessions feel so different? I have already commented on the rhythm of the analyst's interventions early in the session. The tempo of the Kleinian session continues more or less as it started, with the analyst apparently saying about the same amount at about the same intervals throughout the session. We have a sense of work being done in a continuing steady state. With the Freudian analyst it is different. She does not intervene for a long time despite several opportunities. Then there is a partial interpretation, and the tempo picks up significantly toward the end of the session with a sequence of three fuller, much more specific interpretations. This session gives us a sense of trajectory, of an arrival at understanding.

This may look simply like a difference of clinical style and technique. But there is more to it than that. Both analysts work closely in the transference. In fact all of the Freudian analyst's interventions and almost all of the Kleinian analyst's refer to the patient's relationship to or fantasies about the analyst. So the difference in rhythm between the analysts' contributions throughout the session may point to a different attitude to the transference between the two analysts. The Kleinian analyst seems to use the transference to give her a series of snapshots, from moment to moment, of the patient's fantasies and internal object relationships that, from the beginning of the session onward, she is ready to interpret as she observes them. One of the strengths of Kleinian analysis is its alertness to the shifts in the transference throughout the session, so that the most fleeting of affects or fantasies may be caught on the wing and interpreted. What it does not emphasize so much, however, is the slower, longer-term, consistent evolution of the transference in a certain direction. That is what the Freudian analyst is primarily concerned with. She does not make the early interpretations that the Kleinian analyst does because she is using the transference in a different way: not to offer a series of particular insights but cumulatively to arrive at understanding an experience that only develops itself fully over the length of the session.

This difference in *how* the transference is used also shows an important difference in *what* it is being used to interpret. What is there from the beginning is what the patient brings, conscious or unconscious, in his or her own mind: an inner world of fantasy and internal object relationships. For the Kleinian analyst, that is where the oedipal scenario is primarily located and where, to a large extent, her interpretations are directed:

> I felt aware that in the consulting room there was a little girl and somewhere in her mind there is a father and mother together. . . . I said I think it feels

> terrible to feel like the little girl. . . . When that
> happens she switches things around in her mind—
> she imagines herself as the "Daddy," the one who
> gets to be with the "Mummy."

Because this world of internal objects is there in the
patient's mind from the beginning of the session we can interpret it, if the transference will give us the right picture of
it, as early in the session or the analysis as we can grasp it.

What is not there from the beginning is something that
depends for its existence on the development of a mutual
experience, a shared space between patient and analyst. The
Freudian analyst does, of course, interpret the patient's fantasies; an inner world of the patient is certainly being elucidated. But if we look carefully, particularly at the end where
the trajectory of the session issues into overt interpretation,
we see that the interpretative work happens *between* the patient and the analyst, and what is being interpreted is the
reflection of the patient's inner world into the shared space
that they have developed together.

The patient responds to the Freudian analyst's partial
interpretation that "in your mind Stephanie, your mother
and I were all mixed up" by telling her about her husband
coming into the waiting room while he was reading about
beauty contests; he himself makes a connection to when his
father came into the bedroom where he was looking at pictures of brassieres and had an erection. The analyst's next
interpretation, which is about the patient's oedipal guilt,
depends on a previous comment by the patient about the
results of the analysis. The patient then uses the analyst's
interpretation about her husband to explain his guilty feelings toward a colleague and makes his own interpretation
of the unconscious guilt behind his car accident. After the
analyst's next interpretation the patient brings forward his
castration anxiety virtually undisguised in the memory of his

hernia operation. This allows the analyst to make her final and fullest interpretation, but that interpretation still incorporates the patient's own insights about the promotion over his colleague and his excitement about women in the waiting room.

The interpretative work is shared between patient and analyst. Transference interpretations, in this way of working, are not primarily intended to give a view into the patient's world of internal objects so much as to illuminate relationships in that shared analytic space that comprises both inner and outer worlds. They themselves, of course, are also events in that shared space by which it continues to grow and develop.

I have compared these two sessions at some length because we can discern in them a subtle but fundamental difference. I have avoided being too exact about differences among the groups in the British Society because doing so can so easily be misleading. In the Kleinian session, however, I have been pointing to something that is a distinctively Kleinian way of working: the evenly continuing use of a fluctuating transference to allow the analyst to direct interpretations to the patient's fantasy world of internal object relationships. The Freudian analyst, in contrast, illustrates the evolving use of a more progressively developing transference to allow interpretations of what is happening, both in fantasy and reality, in an analytic space that is shared between patient and analyst. Such an approach is more characteristic of the Freudian and Independent groups.

All analysts work by the patient's free associations. One analyst may track those associations as closely as possible to extract the maximum understanding from them. Another, following at a somewhat greater distance, may help the patient feel more freedom of movement and so make a freer, more experimental use of the analytic situation. If we look again at the Independent session we can see this freedom on the patient's part in a rather particular form. The Independendent analyst writes, in his commentary after the clinical material, that "to the end, she was able to challenge and disagree." At the beginning the analyst describes clearly the antagonistic challenging attitude that his patient brought to the analysis. The words "to the end" seem to imply that this attitude continued unabated. The example he actually gives from another session, however, has quite a different quality. He interprets the patient's remark about her baby being a poor little thing without a father as a reference to the analysis being a poor little thing without the analyst. The patient corrects him with her own perception of the analysis as a bouncing baby. This is not a challenge, but constructive disagreement, the use of the analyst's misperception to assert her own point of view. Interestingly there are two examples of constructive disagreement in the session that he presents.

*Pt*:  I want to say to you "Didn't we do well?" But I also feel nothing has changed. I'm still the same person I always was.

*An*: Perhaps you are saying, "Haven't we done well to avoid change."

*Pt*: That seems silly and wrong, because much *has* changed. But I'm glad I'm still the same person.

Given the description of her early antagonism it is remarkable that the patient can now tell the analyst his comment is silly and wrong without that coming across as hostile. She did not mean what he had thought she meant, and she is telling him he has got it wrong. In this exchange we see her freedom to experiment with using the analyst in a particular way, as someone who can be corrected without antagonism. That itself is one of the things that has changed.

This next exchange also occurs at the end, when she talks about swimming:

*Pt*: I'm glad I had some lessons from the instructor.

*An*: I'm the instructor who helped you to swim.

*Pt*: I don't think you ever instructed me or showed me how to do anything. I feel you are the water.

Again the analyst has got it wrong, and again the patient corrects him and in doing so advances the analytic relationship. It is accepted that wrong interpretations, if recognized and worked through, can still have constructive results. But these comments of the analyst hardly qualify as interpretations. They are more by way of his offering an idea or an image of himself, for the patient to make of it what she will. This is an important, although unobtrusive aspect of the Independent analyst's way of analyzing, which is highlighted when the patient's response is one of disagreement.

The Independents and the Contemporary Freudians both tend to think in terms of an analytic space shared between and explored in partnership by both patient and analyst. The Independent session illustrates an aspect of that process that is particularly characteristic of the Independent group. We might express it by saying that *the analyst is there for the patient to find out what use she needs to make of him.*

The patient's feeling that the analyst was not the instructor but the water itself recalls Balint's (1968, p. 66) example of the fish in the sea: "It is an idle question to ask whether the water in the gills or in the mouth is part of the sea or of the fish." Milner (1987, pp. 99, 103) writes that the analyst must be a "pliable substance" and "malleable" for the patient: something controlled or even created by the patient but also with an autonomy of its own. This willingness to be made use of, and not necessarily in ways that we had expected, is a central aspect of the analytic tradition in which the Independent analyst works. He frames his chapter around the technical issue of termination and uses this patient to illustrate it because her termination was so problematic. Yet with hindsight we can see that this apparently unsatisfactory element in her analysis was the way in which she needed to use it. Accepting that her marriage had ended was so difficult both because of the oedipal distortions in her relationship to a man and because of her mother's constant wish to abandon her.

*An*: I think you are saying that you have accepted that your marriage is at an end.

*Pt*: After sixteen years, almost half with you. I must be a slow learner. . . . Although I set the pace for the several premature terminations they could easily have been viewed later as being abandonment by you, just like all the others. The extra year, and especially its timing, stripped away the scaffolding and negated my favorite stance that I was unloved and unlovable. I think it gave me hope.

An analytic space had been created—not insisted on by the patient nor imposed on her by the analyst, but created by the two of them—in which this strange mode of working through the ending of a relationship could take place, a mode that seems on the face of it to be technically undesirable but that turned out to be what the patient needed. Finally being able to accept the ending of her marriage was her most important achievement; and she could only do that by using the analyst in such an analytically unconventional way, made possible by the analyst's pliable but resilient willingness to be used like that.

Given the context of these case presentations it may seem strange that I have not mentioned theoretical differences among different analytic viewpoints about the Oedipus complex itself. Its timing, for example, is a well-known point of disagreement. Interestingly, however, none of these presentations contains specific early infantile material, nor do the analysts generally link their transference interpretations to very early experience. So that area of controversy is not brought forward. They do, however, show us that to speak of analyzing oedipal material may have a wide range of meanings.

For example, we may try to analyze, by recollection and reconstruction, the historical events in the family during the oedipal period together with the fantasies and anxieties attached to them in the child's and his parents' minds at the time. Or we may interpret how oedipal concerns affect the patient's life today, pointing out oedipal patterns of relating and particularly, of course, picking up oedipal elements in the transference. Or we may be more concerned to use external relationships and what we observe in the transference as pointers to unconscious oedipal fantasies in the internal world of our patients. All three analysts use all three of these approaches. They are interrelated strands in the work of analysis that cannot be separated from each other. Our three presentations show us, nonetheless, the difference of emphasis that different analysts may put on one approach or another.

In the Independent analysis, a good deal of attention is paid to what actually happened in the patient's childhood. Being sent away to relatives, the recollection of her father's "turns," which link with the head-banging and the incontinence, her mother saying every night that her father might die: these actual events and their impact on the patient played a large part in the analysis. The other two strands are present, of course, as well. Oedipal transference manifestations are thoroughly analyzed, and there is no shortage of fantasy, such as that of having caused her father's illness and of an unknown but dreadful failure. But the Independent analyst shows us most clearly of the three the importance of the Oedipal history.

The Freudian analyst's emphasis, as she writes, is on analysis of the here and now, particularly in the transference. The importance of reconstructing the developmental history lies in adding a temporal dimension to this primary insight. It is indicative of this emphasis that she gives us no introductory information about her patient's early history. Her presentation illustrates clearly the analysis of the oedipal triangle in the transference, with the sexual attraction to the analyst brought from the unconscious into consciousness and the corresponding fear of reprisal from the analyst's husband declaring itself. This does bring to the patient's mind childhood memories of his father and mother and of his hernia operation when he was 5. It could be asked whether these memories simply add a temporal dimension to the here-and-now transference experience. Do they not also show how that experience can give the patient fresh access to his own history? Either way, though, the Freudian analyst illustrates with great lucidity this strand in the analysis of oedipal material.

The Kleinian analyst's emphasis is more on the third aspect of oedipal analysis, the internal world of unconscious fantasy, and I have quoted already from her session to illustrate this. For the most part she addresses fantasies currently active in the patient's mind, and the main access to these is by their reflection into the transference. But this merges also into the elucidation of fantasies far back in the past and of memories of the past events to which those fantasies relate. Present and past, fantasy and memory are not always clearly distinguished in this way of analyzing. In the patient's unconscious, of course, they are indeed not distinguished; that is exactly the point. When to enter into the patient's unconscious experience and when to bring the distinctions of the conscious mind to bear in disentangling these confusions is something the analyst is always having to judge. In the Kleinian session we see her doing both. I have given an example already of where she seems to equate present-time fantasy and past memory. In her interpretation of the dream about the student, however, she puts the patient in touch specifically with her childhood feelings of not having a penis and therefore inventing a fantasy "tube" to be close to her mother. She interprets the link between that and the current feelings about the analyst, but in a way that helps the patient separate past from present.

We can find a continuity then between these analysts in what the process of analyzing oedipal material means, but within that continuity there is a difference of emphasis. To some extent that may correspond to an overall difference between the groups in the British Society, but variation among analysts within the groups is very great. Although certain points are characteristic of one group or another, I have deliberately discussed these presentations in a discursive rather than systematic fashion so as to avoid describing group differences in a way that might seem plausible but would really be misleading. These presentations, in any case, are individually rich and varied enough in their own right to show us a thought-provoking diversity of approaches to psychoanalysis.

## References

Balint, M. (1968). *The Basic Fault.* London: Tavistock.

Milner, M. (1987). *The Suppressed Madness of Sane Men: Forty-four Years of Exploring Psychoanalysis.* London: Tavistock.

# 11

## Commentary by John Steiner

"How does a theory look in practice when confronted with oedipal content?" This is the question put to the commentators on the three presentations, and my approach to it is consider the reports under a few simple headings.

### The Setting

As a general rule psychoanalysts pay great attention to the setting, which they see as representative of the attitude of the analyst to his work (Segal 1967). All three analysts took a similar approach. They all saw their patients five times a week in a setting that was constant, generally free from intrusions, and designed to allow analytic work to proceed. They paid close attention to the details of the setting, which means that when the setting was disrupted it readily became apparent and the analyst was able to explore its significance for the patient.

  The constancy of the setting is an important aspect of the containing function of the analysis, and when it breaks down or when the patient is unable to tolerate its limitations, this becomes an important factor to be understood. The fact that the Freudian analyst's husband works in a room next to

her and that his patients use the same waiting room is a factor in the setting that she takes account of and recognizes
has an effect on her patients. In the case described this factor seemed to be particularly relevant to the production of
oedipal material, especially when the patient came early and
had to share the waiting room with an attractive woman who
was collected by his analyst's husband.

In the Kleinian analyst's material the fact that the analyst was three minutes late became a departure from the
normal reliability of the setting and was consequently taken
up as having a significance that the session was used to
explore.

The Independent analyst's patient seemed to find it
difficult to accept the limits that the setting offered her. She
complained that the analyst revealed too little of his feelings,
and she tried to provoke him and to break the frame of the
setting in part by her attempts to find out about him through
extra-analytic inquiries.

I cannot find any theoretical differences between these
three analysts over the question of the setting. Theoretical
views such as those of Eissler on parameters (Eissler 1953)
that suggest that adjustments to the setting are required in
the case of certain patients are perhaps more associated with
the members of the Contemporary Freudian group because
of their greater reliance on ego psychology in their theorizing. The members of the group of Independent Analysts in
contrast sometimes seem to favor a more flexible use of the
setting and are perhaps more ready to make modifications,
such as varying the number of sessions offered per week or
offering longer sessions to accommodate the needs of certain patients. This may be particularly relevant in the case of
patients who have been traumatized or those who tend to
regress (Casement 1985, Winnicott 1965). Kleinian analysts
on the other hand usually set great store on maintaining the
stability of the setting, even in those cases where there is

pressure to alter it such as in the treatment of psychotic and borderline patients (Segal 1967). Both of these views however recognize that an attention to stability and a sensitive need of flexibility are important. Real differences in emphasis among the groups in the British Psychoanalytical Society exist in their attitude to various features of the setting, but also there is a great deal of common ground as is evident from the three presentations.

### Transference and Extratransference Interpretations

All three analysts predominantly interpreted the transference, and all made links to the situation in the patient's childhood on the one hand and to events in their current lives on the other.

In the Freudian analyst's sessions the events in the waiting room were linked to those that took place in the patient's relationship with his wife and also with his colleagues at work, and to the acute embarrassment that he felt had parallels in his memory of childhood when he was caught reading a brochure advertising lingerie. All these instances of similar configurations chiefly dealing with exposure, shame, and humiliation were collected by the analyst and integrated as she related them to what was happening between her and the patient.

In the same way the Independent analyst recognized that the dominant event in his patient's childhood was the chronic illness of her father. She reacted to the analyst's unresponsiveness just as she did to her father's masklike face that gave her no indication of his emotional state. Yet, she also resented her mother's nursing of him and her insistence that he would get worse if she was naughty and noisy. This was relived in the transference as she complained that her analyst was unresponsive and did not show his emotions and as she tried to needle him to get him to respond.

The patient of the Kleinian analyst is also reliving a pattern of object relationships that developed in her childhood. At one point she became irritable and started rubbing the new wallpaper, which she mentioned for the first time. She then described how as a child she had been temporarily moved out of the nursery to a room with similar paper at a time when she was one of three children and her mother was pregnant with the fourth. She made a mess of the wallpaper and also of her bed by spilling some cod-liver oil. Later her mother denied that she would have been angry over this. However, the patient did seem to feel that the present climate of the sessions was a repetition of something going on then, and at this point of the session she clearly did feel in a mess and she expected the analyst to be angry. By interpreting the reliving of these experiences in the transference the Kleinian analyst was able to collect the various episodes and to show a common pattern in them.

Again there seems to be a communality of technique in which the interpretation of transference is given a central role in all three cases. However, there may be differences in the way in which extratransference interpretations are treated. For example the Freudian analyst understands the oedipal themes to involve whole object relations, and she links her patient's humiliation to his relationship with her husband when he is forced to observe him in the waiting room. This is partly in the transference, but also partly outside it, referring to what happens in the waiting room between the patient and the analyst's husband. An alternative or perhaps an additional approach might be to try to collect the feelings in the transference by interpreting the humiliating, castrating figure to be operating in the session as an aspect of the analyst herself. In this way a punitive transference could be recognized that exists alongside the more acceptable supportive transference.

## Enactments in the Transference and
## the "Here and Now"

A major development in British psychoanalysis has arisen from the recognition that the analyst is persuaded to behave in ways that correspond to something going on in the patient. The Sandlers have made important contributions to the theory of the way in which role-relationships are enacted in the analytic situation (Sandler 1976, Sandler and Sandler 1978); this is a point of common ground with those Kleinian analysts who are influenced by the work of Betty Joseph (1981, 1987, 1988). An interest in this theme requires a detailed attention to subtle nuances in the patient–analyst interaction during the session and leads to a type of analysis that concentrates on the here-and-now.

Both the Sandlers and Betty Joseph have recognized the ways in which patients nudge and prod the analyst in order to create a particular situation in the transference. Sandler (1976) describes how an internal situation involving relations between the self and objects becomes actualized in the relationship with the analyst, who is then led to enact an infantile role relationship. As a counterpart to Freud's free-floating attention he points out that the analyst has to have a free-floating responsiveness and that the analyst's reactions as well as his thoughts and feelings contribute to his countertransference. Joseph takes this theme further and shows how it is through enactments that the analyst is drawn into playing a role in the patient's phantasy and as a result is used as part of his defensive system.

All three analysts seem to be aware of the pressure on them to act in particular ways, and they used this to varying degrees in their understanding of the transference. The Independent analyst, for example, interprets the way his patient repeatedly knocked him down and then built him up, and he connected this with the configuration in her family, namely that she wanted to look after him as she had wanted to look after her father and that she first had to make him weak and could then in phantasy replace her mother and build him up. This formulation helped him contain her anxiety about stopping and also his own anxiety about the feelings she provoked in him. In addition, I had the impression that the repeated building up and slapping down drew the analyst into a sadomasochistic relationship that was impossible to resist and very difficult to interpret.

Similarly the Kleinian analyst was aware of the way in which her patient fails to mention things that impinge on her and that probably have great significance for her. This is the case with the new wallpaper in the consulting room and also with the fact that the analyst was three minutes late for the session. However, when the analyst repeatedly tried to draw attention to the significance of her lateness, she was enacting something that I suspect she had been unconsciously nudged into doing. The patient could feel blocked by traffic because she felt that her analyst was preoccupied with her lateness, and she pointedly declined to help remove the blockage by refusing to discuss this issue.

The Freudian analyst is very aware of what is happening in the here and now of the analytic session, but she too is inevitably nudged into playing a role in the patient's defensive organization. It seems clear that the transference had become highly eroticized and that the prevailing feeling in both patient and analyst was a positive one linked to a recognition of the progress that had been made. This reality was a factor used by the patient to prod the analyst to enact the role of an indulgent wife. In this session she appeared to avoid upsetting him and joined in the reassurance that he need not feel bad about his impotence. The negative punitive feelings that chiefly involve humiliation of various kinds are present but split off and ascribed to the patient's father and to the analyst's husband.

This kind of enactment in the transference is not only inevitable, but through its analysis can become a convincing way by which both patient and analyst may gain an understanding of the mental mechanisms involved in the patient's object relationships.

According to Gill (1979), it is important to interpret the current reality that emerges in the transference, but in a comment on his work (Steiner 1984) I have argued that it is not always easy to recognize what this current reality is. The countertransference is usually to a large extent unconscious, and it is only through analytic work that what has been going on may become apparent to the analyst. In some cases the patient will eventually help the analyst in this task, but not all patients will be so obliging, and support from a third object outside the patient–analyst couple may be vital.

## The Timing of Interpretations

One difference among the three analysts was the readiness with which they verbalized the thoughts and observations they made. This is most evident in the Freudian analyst's material since she reported making formulations about what she believed was going on and then deciding not to interpret them to the patient. The Kleinian analyst, in contrast, seemed to be giving voice to her thoughts much earlier. Perhaps this is a group difference, but it may also be a function of the style and character of the analyst and also of the patient. It is easier to bring more cooperative and less disturbed patients into the analytic process as partners, whereas with more disturbed patients it is necessary to consider what the patient is capable of assimilating.

It is possible to find theoretical reason for these differences, but they are also a factor of the personality of the
analyst and perhaps are influenced by tradition and fashion.
Some analysts with some patients prefer to share more of
what they are thinking as it is happening. With other patients
it may be dangerous to do this.

A related issue concerns the degree of explicit references to primitive images of body parts and sexual acts. Such
images were so explicit in the material from the Freudian
analyst's patient that she perhaps did not want to embarrass
him by picking up concrete fellatio phantasies and linking
them to the mucus resulting from her cold, even though these
linkages were clearly conscious or nearly so in her patient.
In this respect there has been a change in the style of Kleinian
work that has brought it more into line with the way Contemporary Freudians practice. We are now more concerned
about recognizing the motives and movements in the transference and have tended to be more cautious about references to explicit sexual material (Spillius 1983). Perhaps this
is an example of how the groups have influenced each other
in the British Society.

## The Appearance of Oedipal Themes

It is perhaps over the theory of the Oedipus complex that
we might expect theoretical differences among the groups
to be most evident. Melanie Klein recognized early stages of
the Oedipus complex beginning soon after birth and becoming well established by the onset of the depressive position
in the first half of the first year. Kleinian analysts might discern primitive versions of the oedipal configuration in various aspects of the case material presented, particularly when
a triangular configuration was present. A Contemporary
Freudian analyst would be more inclined to consider oedi-

pal phantasies to arise later between the third and fifth year of life and to conceptualize them in terms of more mature whole object relationships. Indeed the Freudian analyst confirms this view by telling us that the task of finding an oedipal session was far from easy. Here she is clarifying that in common with most British analysts she finds that many of her patients are operating at a primitive borderline level that she views as preoedipal. In this way she does not consider everything triangular to be oedipal, and it is this conceptualization that leads her to place more emphasis on the more mature elements of the Oedipus complex that her patient illustrated so nicely.

Partly this is a problem of nomenclature, as the Freudian analyst is certainly concerned with early primitive relationships, particularly two-person relationships that dominate the transference in borderline and psychotic patients. Certainly we all agree that the way the infant has negotiated the preoedipal two-person relationship profoundly affects the impact of the Oedipus situation. Nevertheless real differences exist, both in our views of part-object oedipal configurations and in our propensity to interpret even mature versions of the oedipal configuration in terms of underlying primitive part-object phantasies.

The issue of the role played by the analyst's husband in the Freudian analysis can serve as an illustration of how oedipal configurations can be viewed. In his actual appearance in the waiting room he represents a whole object aspect of the mature Oedipus complex, whereas as an internal figure projected onto the analyst in the transference he can, in addition, be seen to represent a split-off part of the analyst that was less reassuring and less friendly to the patient's oedipal enactments.

Perhaps a Kleinian analyst would also have given more weight to the primal scene configuration created by the patient's actual encounter with the analyst's husband and the phantasies that are stimulated by it. Humiliation and shame played such a large part in the patient's experience, which often arises when the patient's narcissism is wounded as a result of having his oedipal enactments exposed. Such narcissistic wounding tends to involve an observing, judging, and often condemning object who exposes the pretensions of the overly narcissistic child. If the infant has established a good relationship with the primary object he can tolerate the emergence of the third object without undue shame. If, however, the infant, either through his own omnipotence or encouraged by his mother, develops too strong a narcissistic conviction that he is preferred to the father, then the humiliation and exposure can be devastating.

With the Kleinian presentation, the analyst's lateness was seen to represent an oedipal configuration in the sense that the patient would see it as the intrusion of a third object into the time that had been allocated to her. Subsequently as the analyst repeatedly interpreted the lateness, her preoccupation with it was an additional factor that may have come to represent a third object lodged in the analyst's mind.

It was this oedipal theme that made the early parts of the session so stormy and difficult. Later the patient and analyst were in much better contact and more able to face painful reality together. The patient became sad, thinking "What is the use?," and recalled what is was like playing with the older girls next door and that she had hurt her shoulder as they swung her round by the arm. With the establishment of better contact I believe the patient was able to tell the analyst that she felt injured and hurt by the way she has been treated by her. At first she wanted to get rid of the hurt by getting rid of the third object in the oedipal configuration in order to create an ideal romantic couple. Subsequently through the sensitivity of the analyst she is able to share her sense of sadness and to recognize the painful reality of her relationship with her.

Another area of theoretical difference concerns the role played by castration threats and anxieties. We can look at this theme in the Freudian analysis when the patient described how his indulgent mother was frightened of his father and would punish him only at his father's insistence. This led the analyst to interpret that the patient was afraid that her husband would resent the good relationship that the patient had developed with her. The patient responded with an account of the colleague who was resentful at his promotion, and he described the bash to the wing of his car as he drove out of his driveway. The Freudian analyst again picks up a positive wish in her patient. She interprets that although he is concerned with rivalry and aggression he also wants to make peace. The patient enthusiastically agrees and describes the hernia scar that seemed to stand for the punishment that his mother would administer at his father's insistence if he was not ready to make this peace. Finally the analyst makes a classical oedipal transference interpretation linking the patient's current fear of her husband with his earlier fear of castration, and she suggests that this fear was triggered by his promotion.

Here a Kleinian analyst might have been more concerned with the aggression and with the fear of punishment and humiliation. Although the patient undoubtedly feels stronger overall, in this particular session he does not seem to feel promoted in any realistic way as a result of his achievement in relation to his analyst. Another view would be that his promotion over the head of his colleague makes him excited so that he becomes manic, smashing his car and becoming sexually impotent and infantile. He then turns to the reassurance of his indulgent mother, wife, and analyst.

It may be relevant here to contrast the classical theory of the dissolution of the Oedipus complex with the alternative derived from the work of Klein. In the classical version the child's challenge to his father is thwarted by the reality of the castration threat, which leads to a renunciation of the primary object and an identification with the threatening father. In this type of resolution the patient identifies with this father and through his strength is able to tackle his adult sexual roles. It leaves him, however, treating his own sons in the same threatening way in which his father treated him. It is a victory for the father and leads to shame and humiliation, which may remain as sources of resentment and a desire for vengeance.

Simultaneously an alternative scenario exists in the unconscious, which results from the initial excited triumph over the father. If the child enacts this scenario in phantasy he eventually comes to realize that it not only leaves him bereft of a father but that it also leaves his mother bereft, and this realization can confront him with the need to face his depression and guilt, which arise as a result of the oedipal crime. An analysis of this situation leads to depression and despair, and it is only if these feelings are worked through that the move toward reparation and forgiveness can begin. Such a depressive solution to the Oedipus situation exists alongside the persecutory solution that Freud described and the Freudian analyst has identified in her material. It may have been represented in the session by the fact that the analyst was not well and the patient was sufficiently worried to think that he perhaps should have spared her and not come. He may have been afraid that he had hurt her and that his enactments with his wife and with his car had made her depressed. Because of his evasion of guilt and responsibility for what he had done in phantasy, he could not embark on the task of making reparation and instead had used her indulgence to reassure himself that his sexuality was not damaging.

Both the depressive and the paranoid solution to the Oedipus conflict are important, and both have to be interpreted eventually. Of course, both ways of interpreting the material can be taken to excess, and that is why it is so important to listen to the patient and use his reactions to monitor how the analyst's work is being experienced. The analyst can then adapt his approach to take account of what his patient is telling him.

We can look at the same question in the Independent's material. His patient was indeed terrified of ending her analysis, and she had little belief that she could cope with mourning and loss. Yet, she made more use of her analysis than she was prepared to admit, and from it she had learned a great deal, not only about her own sadism and the reasons for it but also about her analyst's capacity to suffer her cruelty and to cope with it. Nevertheless she went on until the end of her analysis attempting to achieve an oedipal fulfillment rather than to face an oedipal loss with the blow to her omnipotence that it would entail. Even in the last session she seemed to be using negation to deal with her grief at the loss of the analysis, saying that it was *not* a poor little thing having lost its father, but a bouncy baby.

### Conclusions

It is a pleasure to comment on material that I think is fairly representative of work in the British Psycho-Analytical Society. These reports do show differences in the basic approach of the three analysts and no doubt some of these differences are due to a different theoretical base. At the same time many other factors differentiate the three individuals, including differences in personality and cultural background. In fact not one of the three analysts was born or educated in Britain. The Freudian analyst comes from Geneva, the Independent analyst from Dublin, and the Kleinian analyst from Los Angeles. This is quite typical of the British Psycho-Analytical Society, which has been host to many analysts from

Central Europe and which continues to provide a professional home to colleagues from a wide range of countries and cultures.

Finally it seems worth noting the difficult position I found myself in when responding to the request to comment on these presentations. The first thing that struck me was that this apparently straightforward task was far from simple and involved me in complex conflicts that introduced aspects of the Oedipus situation itself. If I am asked to witness and make judgments on the relationship of the analyst and his patient, the analyst and his theory, or the analyst and his group, I am immediately placed in the position of an observer who is part voyeur. I have earlier emphasized the importance of a third object who can help the analyst by providing another point of view, and it is relevant to point out that this situation that can be so important and supportive also has its dangers.

It is inevitable that the third object is not part of the relationship between the patient and the analyst and is invited to participate in phantasy, to put himself in the place of the patient or of the analyst, and to imagine what his experience would be. This is a situation where the observer will be tempted to act out, to imagine that he knows what is going on and to adopt a moral stance. It is always difficult to remain outside the primal couple, and we may participate by too intense or too biased an identification with one or other of the participants. This type of projective identification allows us to acquire an empathic understanding using the phantasy of how we would feel in the situation of one or other of the participants, but it can be misleading if we assume that we know what either of them is going through. We can become partisan and try to protect the patient from a bad analyst or vice versa to defend the analyst in an overprotective way. Here too other motives such as rivalry and prejudice can easily enter disguised in various ways and may lead to intrusive and disturbing oedipal enactments. In order to understand properly we must return to our own identity as an observer to listen, to watch, and to be aware as much as we can of our own motives, and this is usually only possible in the context of an ongoing relationship.

The dangers are greater in the present setting where I am not invited to comment by the authors but by the editors, and the task set me could easily encourage partisanship since it involves not simply a third point of view of one patient–analyst couple but a comparison of three such couples. To write a commentary for publication can easily lead the commentator to become involved in rivalry that may be divisive and prejudiced.

Many of the quarrels that have developed among different schools of thought are ugly and divisive, and much pain is created, as can be seen by anyone who has read an account of the controversial discussions (King and Steiner 1991). Fortunately we have learned to live with this situation, and despite periodic tensions and conflicts we do manage to survive as a united society. However, like oedipal conflicts, the tensions and rivalries that such competing ideologies give rise to are wasteful and unproductive, even if they are unavoidable. This is particularly true when, as in oedipal conflicts, primitive part-object relationships dominate.

In fact most of the tension arises from political allegiances and loyalties and not theoretical differences. The latter can be worked through, provided enough time and trouble are taken to understand the other person's point of view. In fact the three authors of the present contributions are well known for the way they understand and respect the work of colleagues in the other groups, and I hope that this is the example that the reader will want to emulate. It requires each of us to face painful issues about ourselves and our relationships, and when these are too difficult we will no doubt continue to deal with conflict through infantile means.

# References

Casement, P. (1985). *On Learning from the Patient.* London: Routledge.

Eissler, K. R. (1953). The effect of the structure of the ego on psychoanalytic technique. *Journal of the American Psychoanalytic Association* 1:104–143.

Gill, M. M. (1979). The analysis of transference. *Journal of the American Psychoanalytic Association* 27:263–288.

Joseph, B. (1981). Towards the experiencing of psychic pain. In *Do I Dare Disturb the Universe? A Memorial to W. R. Bion,* ed. J. S. Grotstein. Beverly Hills: Caesura Press. Reprinted in *Psychic Equilibrium and Psychic Change: Selected Papers of Betty Joseph,* ed. M. Feldman and E. B. Spillius. London: Routledge, 1989.

—— (1987). Projective identification: some clinical aspects. In *Projection, Identification, Projective Identification,* ed. J. Sandler. New York: International Universities Press. Reprinted in *Psychic Equilibrium and Psychic Change: Selected Papers of Betty Joseph,* ed. M. Feldman and B. Spillius. London: Routledge, 1989.

—— (1988). Object relations in clinical practice. *Psychoanalytic Quarterly,* 57:626–42. Reprinted in *Psychic Equilibrium and Psychic Change: Selected Papers of Betty Joseph,* ed. M. Feldman and E. B. Spillius. London: Routledge, 1989.

King, P., and Steiner, R. (1991). *The Freud-Klein Controversies 1941–45.* London: Routledge.

Sandler, J. (1976). Countertranference and role-responsiveness. *International Review of Psycho-Analysis* 3:43–47.

Sandler, J., and Sandler, A. M. (1978). On the development of object relationships and affects. *International Journal of Psycho-Analysis* 59:285–296.

Segal, H. (1967). Melanie Klein's Technique. In *Psycho-analytic Techniques,* ed. B. B. Wolman. New York: Basic

Books. Reprinted in *The Work of Hanna Segal.* New York: Jason Aronson, 1981.

Spillius, E. B. (1983). Some developments from the work of Melanie Klein. *International Journal of Psycho-Analysis* 64:321–332.

Steiner, J. (1984). Some reflections on the analysis of transference: a Kleinian view. *Psycho-Analytic Inquiry,* 4:443–463.

Winnicott, D. W. (1965). *The Maturational Processes and the Facilitating Environment.* London: Hogarth.

# V

# SYNTHESIS AND CONCLUSION

# 12

# Pluralism and Convergence in the Clinical Setting

*DANIEL HILL*
*CAROLE GRAND*

## Introduction

After an initial period of theory expansion and diversification, psychoanalysis has entered a period of consolidation. There is a convergence—an interpenetrating of ideas among theories and an integration of theories—that is taking place both formally and informally. The driving force for this convergence is the very theoretical pluralism produced by the first one hundred years of psychoanalysis.

It is impossible for contemporary psychoanalysts to avoid the strains of the theoretical pluralism that marks their intellectual world. For those entering the field, it is the hydra with which one struggles in forming a professional identity. Later it influences choices about institutions with which to be affiliated, about how one practices, and about whom one has for colleagues. However, these choices are no longer what they once were. The position that "the theory to which I subscribe and the way I practice is correct and the alternatives are wrong" has become less and less tenable. At the least, each school of thought and each practitioner is forced to take into account the most compelling ideas of their competitors. Those drawn to orthodoxy of whatever theoretical persuasion have been softened by a variety of factors including a history of unscientific and unproductive arguing, an erosion of ideas that once seemed like bedrock, the general acceptance (even among the orthodox) of ideas that once seemed heretical, the lack of any outcome studies that give preference to one theory over another, insistent arguments that metapsychologies are superfluous and/or metaphorical, and, finally, now, compelling integrations and syntheses. Postmodernism has not spared psychoanalysis.

This study has been an instance of using pluralism to advance our thinking about the clinical situation while at the same time assessing the status of psychoanalytic thought in the context of that pluralism. Before this project we organized, over a three-year period, seventeen Analysts-in-Session (AIS) Workshops in which leading theorists and practitioners, identified as Freudians, presented single sessions of an ongoing case (one presentation per evening, unlike the three in one day of the conference that led to this book). The presentations and the formal and informal discussions that surrounded the AIS workshops were an education in the range of diversity of so-called classical analysts. "So-called" because there is no monolithic body of ideas, and there is little left of the orthodoxy that enforced allegiance to fantasies of them; there are few shibboleths or comments about not being a "real *P*sychoanalyst."

The AIS Workshops took place at New York University's Postdoctoral Program in Psychoanalysis and Psychotherapy, which, like the British Society, houses several psychoanalytic groups. (In the case of NYU the groups function under the rubrics of Freudian, Interpersonal, Relational, and Nonaligned.) Again, like the British Society, NYU Postdoc functions as a microcosm of the field with all its theoretical arguments, politics, social pressures, confusion, and intellectual vitality. From this vantage, the NYU Postdoc training and affiliation, the experiences with the workshops, and the conference focusing on the British Psycho-Analytical Society, we have seen not only the manifold changes taking place among

Freudians but also among practitioners of other psychoanalytic identities.

An unsettled and unsettling theoretical pluralism is a central component of the environment in which psychoanalysis is now conceived and practiced. It acts as a tension eliciting the development of new ideas and their integration into existing theories. By asking the commentators to compare and contrast the work of the three different authors representing the three different orientations of the British Psycho-Analytical Society we made pluralism *the* context of this project. Within that context one is likely to encounter the unresolved discussion that continues in response to Wallerstein's (1990) proposal that there is a clinical theory that acts as a "common ground" shared by all psychoanalysts. By asking that the authors choose a session to present in which oedipal material was a central issue, we also provided an opportunity to see how some of the most thoughtful members of the field now view material that has historically held center stage. We believed that it was time to look again at the oedipal constellation in order to ascertain, in this limited way, the place it held in current thinking. Finally, as discussed in the preface, the project intended to use pluralism as a catalyst for creativity and new thinking.

Although working independently, the authors of individual sessions and the commentators collectively contributed to the common aim of cross-theoretical study. The bulk of this chapter is devoted to summarizing, integrating, and occasionally synthesizing the results of their work. Obviously, we cannot hope to include all that is valuable. We have chosen to focus on aspects that move debates forward, on new ideas, and on methodologies that will aid future cross-theoretical studies. Along with these yields, the project illuminated both the diversity and the convergences in the field, and it is these that provide a starting point for our summary.

In the past one read psychoanalytic material in the context of knowing whether the writer was a Freudian, Kleinian, and so on. However, as can be seen in the responses of both the authors and the commentators, theoretical boundaries have been blurred. Moreover, the old labels have lost much of their original meanings. Indeed, for many psychoanalysts, they now mark social and political fault lines more than clear-cut borders among collections of ideas. In attempting to appreciate the ideas put forth in the previous chapters we did not find it particularly useful to think of the writer according to the traditional taxonomy. Rather it was preferable to have a way of locating them according to their "response to pluralism." Toward this end we have attempted to schematize the various ways of responding to pluralism. This scheme serves as a lens both to focus our thoughts and to map those of the authors and commentators.

### Responses to Pluralism

To understand the effects of pluralism one must look carefully at what is meant by the term *convergence. There are different types of convergence, and the kind of convergence one constructs is a function of one's response to pluralism.* We have already offered a two-part definition for convergence: (1) an interpenetration of ideas among theories and (2) an integration of theories. Convergence can be further understood if we look at its manifestations.

Convergence takes different forms as a function of three distinct responses to pluralism. Traditionally, there is a *particularistic response* in which one takes a side in the dialectics of pluralism, promoting, modifying, and defending the particular theory to which one subscribes. It is a formal response with careful attention paid to maintaining the integrity of the theory. For the particularist, pluralism provides an atmosphere of lively debate. The fruit of the particularist response is the continuing evolution of each of the particular theories in response to the dialectics (Schafer 1990). In some instances the theory assimilates ideas. In other cases, ideas are dropped or revised to accommodate valid criticism and new data. Although the accommodations and assimilations of the Freudian groups have been the most often observed and articulated (see for example Greenberg and Mitchell 1983), particularist strategies are equally characteristic of the other schools of thought.

In Chapter 10, Parsons has commented that the schools of thought differ according to what they emphasize. Pine (1991) has argued elsewhere that they all attempt to encompass the full range of mental life and that they differ according to assumptions of motivational primacy. Certainly each theoretical position has been influenced by the thinking of the other schools of thought. In this volume we have explicit evidence of the influence of pluralism on particularists in the introduction of the Freudian analyst and in the commentary of Burgner (Chapter 9) and Ellman (Chapter 6). And, we can see it writ large in the new names adopted by two of the groups in the British Society—*Contemporary* Freudians and *Modern* Kleinians.

Another form of convergence is found in the *universalist responses* of Wallerstein (1990, 1992) and Pine (1990). A universalist attempts to find truth in commonalities that all psychoanalysts endorse. Wallerstein (1992) argues that there is a clinical theory to which all psychoanalysts subscribe, regardless of their metapsychology. He calls this the "common ground" of psychoanalysis. Moreover, he argues that the metapsychologies are "large scale explanatory metaphors, or symbolisms, which we use to give a sense of coherence and closure to our psychological understanding and therefore to our psychoanalytic interventions" and "articles of faith . . . beyond the realm of empirical study and scientific process" (p. 56).

Pine has taken a slightly less radical, but no less creative approach. He has treated an array of psychoanalytic theories as a kind of common wisdom from which he distills four essences—four organizations of mind and a corresponding set of theoretical models for clinical practice. He refers to these—both the actual organizations of mind and the theoretical models derived from them—as the "psychologies" of drive, ego, object relations, and self experience and argues that they encompass the full range of mental life as psychoanalysis has come to know it.

Finally, and perhaps most commonly, there is a third response to pluralism that takes place informally and is found in the *eclecticism* of the Independents of both the British Psycho-Analytical Society and the NYU Postdoctoral Program. In all likelihood it is also the response of many if not most practitioners influenced by the pressures of the work as they face patients who do not fit neatly into the theoretical framework in which they were trained, but seem instead to fit the models of other points of view. The position is stated most eloquently in Burgner's opening statement (Chapter 9). A member of the Contemporary Freudian group, she refers to it as a disclaimer providing her a measure of freedom from the constraints of categorization.

> It is important for me, as a practicing child and adult analyst, to know that I have a substantial and accessible body of theory. But it has always seemed of equal importance that I should be capable of an analytic stance in the consulting room that does not lean too heavily and too automatically upon any one analytic formulation. In such a desirable analytic mental set, John Keats's (1817) definition of

"negative capability" is relevant: "that is when a man is capable of being in uncertainties, mysteries, doubts, without any irritable reaching after fact and reason" (p. 72). My endeavor not to be too dependent or attached to any one theory is, in part, connected with an awareness that the theories we are taught, the theories we gradually become most attracted to, the theories that inform our understanding of our daily clinical work, practically all of these are in essence conceptual models of the mind, metaphors that, as Wallerstein (1988) writes, have been created "in order to satisfy our variously conditioned needs for closure and coherence and overall theoretical understanding" (p. 15).

In the atmosphere of pluralism, and, for some, in the knowledge that no metaphor is complete, the response is to pick and choose from among the full array of ideas put forth by the competing theories. The results are personal theories (Modell 1994) with which to work in clinical-life-as-lived. In the past this was done furtively to avoid the political and economic ramifications. However, increasingly this informal and organic response comes with a measure of pride about having carved out an autonomous identity free of the constraints of implicit and explicit dictates about "correct" thinking.

Figure 12–1 schematizes the responses to pluralism. We have depicted a continuum within the particularistic response ranging from the orthodoxy of those who resist changes in a particular theory to those who are actively attempting to modify and expand a particular theory by assimilating ideas contributed from other schools of thought and accommodating well-founded criticism. Within the universalist response we have depicted the two approaches that have emerged thus far.

**Figure 12–1.** RESPONSES TO PLURALISM

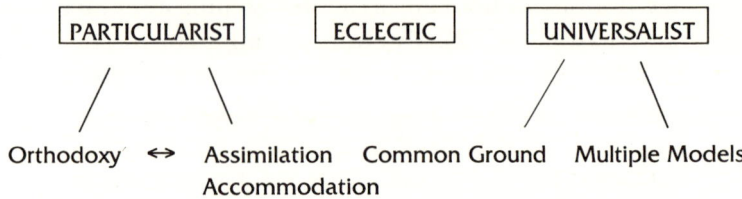

The Determinants of Clinical Processes

*Metapsychology and Characteristics of Analysts
as Influences on Clinical Process*

Wallerstein's proposal of clinical theory as a psychoanalytic common ground and the controversy that continues to swirl around it provide the context for comments about the influence of metapsychology on clinical process. The controversy hinges on the linkage or lack thereof of metapsychology and technique. If Wallerstein is correct that our metapsychologies are but metaphors and that we share a common ground in our clinical theory, then there is a disjuncture between the varying metapsychologies and the invariant technical common ground. In response to the presentations in this study, the controversy emerges primarily in the commentary about the timing of interventions.

Four of the commentators take up the issue of timing, or, as Parsons refers to it, "the tempo" of the session. Attention is paid both to when the Kleinian analyst begins her interventions (immediately) and to the frequency of her interventions (often), in contrast to the Freudian analyst and the Independent analyst who wait until well into the session and offer interventions less frequently.

Let us begin with the comments of Wallerstein (Chapter 8). His thinking is subtle on the differences among the presentations. He notes that the Freudian analyst's introductory remarks "can represent a convergence in thinking of all three of the main theoretical streams in the British psychoanalysis." At the same time, he sees a definite difference in "conception and technique" among the presentations from representatives of those streams. Finally, for Wallerstein, these differences do not reflect differences that accrue from how a Contemporary Freudian or Modern Kleinian, or Independent analyst inevitably practices, but rather from differences in the analytic style or temperament of the individual analysts.

These are seeming contradictions. Moreover, at first glance, some of these notions do not seem to fit with his view that there is a clinical common ground. However, for Wallerstein, none of this is contradictory because he differentiates among four independent factors: that the metapsychologies are converging, that there are differences in the clinical processes reported by the presenters, that there is a common clinical theory, and that the obvious differences in the clinical processes are a function of the characteristics of the analysts.

Wallerstein is critical of the tempo of the Kleinian analyst's session in comparison to that of the Freudian and Independent analyst, but argues that there is nothing in the theory itself that drives this difference in technique. "It is easy enough to call these different interpretive styles typically— or again stereotypically—Freudian or Kleinian, but to me there is nothing inherent in ego psychological or in Kleinian theory that requires these differences in approach; that is, to me, they are not theory-driven or theory-determined." He does not deny the "theory-linked differences in choice of interventions and in the style and language of interventions." However, for Wallerstein, the differences in timing are products of the analysts' personal style expressed within an adherence to a universal clinical theory. And in keeping with the unifying spirit of his argument, he observes that

> The overarching commonality of our clinical ap-
> proach to the phenomena of the analytic interac-
> tion in the consulting room transcends both our
> individual difference of style and temperament as
> unique people and the conceptual differences
> of our theoretical explanatory frameworks, and
> brings us together as identifiably all psychoanalysts
> doing the common work of psychoanalysis in com-
> parable enough ways."

Ellman (Chapter 6) is also critical of the tempo the Kleinian
analyst displays in the session she presents. However, in stark
contrast to Wallerstein and while being careful not to over-
state the case, he argues that technique is inevitably and to
varying degrees linked to theory and that it should be. He
proposes that it is the Kleinian emphasis on projective identification that is responsible for the Kleinian analyst's style.
Although he does not elaborate on this point, the implication is clearly that although each of the groups keeps a steady
eye on the here-and-now of the transference and uses it clinically to understand the patient's dynamics and to give the
analytic process an emotional vitality, it is the Kleinians who
are overly focused on it. For example, Betty Joseph tells us,

> I think that this process is so powerful and yet so
> subtle that it makes it essential for the analyst, first
> of all, to focus attention on what is going on and
> how he or she is being pushed or pulled emotion-
> ally to experience or behave in various ways. And
> what the patient says, in itself, of course extremely
> important, has to be seen within the framework of
> what the patient does. This, of course, implies that
> there is always an object relationship in the consult-
> ing room and that our first task is to be aware of
> the active nature of the relationship. [1988, p. 630]

She goes on to discuss, ". . . how focusing primarily on the object relationship that the patient lives out in the room can help us to listen analytically and therefore to sort out the nature of his immediate conflicts and his method of dealing with them" (p. 631).

Ellman makes his argument for the influence of meta-psychology more fully when he takes aim (see below) at the Freudian analyst's assertion that the infantile neurosis has all but been abandoned as a clinically useful concept among Contemporary Freudians.

Pine (Chapter 7) and Parsons (Chapter 10) also note the difference in tempo between the Kleinian analyst and the other presenters, but both take the position that there are too many uncontrolled variables affecting the process to make a definitive judgment about the relative effect of meta-psychology on technique. Interestingly, Parsons does go on to attribute the differences in tempo to the school of thought to which one subscribes.[1] He does not, however, go so far as to say that the differences are entirely theory driven, but states his impression that there are differences in what the groups

---

1. Richards and Richards (in press) have summarized a controversy in the British Psycho-Analytical Society concerning what is being called tempo in this study. "One issue that divided Kleinians from ego psychologists was the number and depth of interpretations thought appropriate for an hour (King and Steiner 1991). At that time, Kleinians gave many more than the followers of Anna Freud. Recently, Levine (1992) reported a discussion in which modern Kleinians, Segal and Etchegoyen, give no more interpretations in an hour than the modern ego psychologist Weinshel. But not all modern Kleinians agree on this point. Racker (1968) has taken Klein's idea that interpretations must be offered at the point of urgency to mean that more is better. Etchegoyen (1991) has taken it to mean that interpretations are useful only when they become urgent."

emphasize. What is responsible for the differences in emphasis is left open to question. Pine, in contrast, concludes that "there is nothing in these three presentations that permits me to separate out group differences." In contrast to Ellman and in keeping with Wallerstein, Pine concludes that "none of the presentations seemed particularly theory-driven; each seemed to reveal the responsiveness of the analyst to what the patient brought in."

This alignment and the differences among the commentators are most understandable when one considers that Pine and Wallerstein have universalist responses to pluralism, that Burgner is eclectic, that Ellman responds from a particularist point of view, and that Parsons and Steiner are commenting on particularism. The universalist, interested in the common determinants of clinical process does not see group differences that accrue from different metapsychologies. Parsons, who takes a neutral position, notes the group differences and strives to appreciate the value of each. Finally, the particularist, supporting a preference for one metapsychology over others, and the eclectic, valuing a variety of ideas, emphasize the differences. This position is especially evident when Ellman responds to the Freudian analyst's comments about the place of the infantile neurosis in the work of Contemporary Freudians.

Ellman (Chapter 6) takes issue with the Freudian analyst's introductory statement that the infantile neurosis is practically "never used; rather we tend from the beginning of the analysis to think of transference manifestations in the here and now of the session." He couches his criticism in terms of the present and past unconscious (Sandler and Sandler 1994). He argues that her interpretations refer to both the past and present unconscious, and as is inevitable, that the former are dealt with through reconstruction. He then goes on to demonstrate that in the Freudian analyst's presentation there are "clear example(s) of reconstruction based on certain theoretical ideas about the early form of the patient's neurosis." For Ellman, Freudian theory *requires* reconstructive interventions, and in stating that she interprets the present unconscious rather than the past unconscious the Freudian analyst fails to notice that both are woven together in her interventions. With this, Ellman's particularist position takes shape—theory is or should be linked to technique, and the past unconscious is as much a part of an analysis based in (contemporary) Freudian theory as the present unconscious. According to Ellman, the Freudian analyst believes she has gotten away from the use of the infantile neurosis, but as a subscriber to Freudian metapsychology, she cannot.

Based on the divergent conclusions about the effects of metapsychology versus the effects of the characteristics of analysts, it seems as though Pine's and Parson's observation has merit. That is, that the number of uncontrolled variables makes it impossible to come to a definitive conclusion about group differences. Certainly no consensus has been reached in this study, and given the lack of empirical means to test the problem, it would seem that the debate could continue indefinitely without resolution. It is, however, hard to dismiss the common observation that there are different clinical styles associated with each of the different groups. (Parsons seems to have based his conclusions on this and his own perceptions of group differences.)

All three British commentators acknowledge differences in clinical technique that they describe as emanating from the three different theoretical bases. Parson's position has already been mentioned and is discussed again below. Burgner (Chapter 9), although she points out that one needs "to bear in mind that there is considerable variation and discrepancy in approach between members of any one group in the society," also tells us that "three analysts from different groups within the British Society would inevitably use psychoanalytic concepts differently in their clinical work. . . . Yet, the divergence and, for that matter, the convergence of conceptualization in the three presented cases are seen more in technique than in conceptualization . . . in terms of timing of interpretations, and the amount said to their patients . . . in the maintenance of a transferential emphasis as opposed to the additional and judicious use of construction and reconstruction in bringing an eventual coherence to transference interpretations."

Burgner also sees the work of the Independent analyst as "different again in terms of technique, apparently intervening regularly in response to what the patient says."

Steiner (Chapter 11) discusses the same issues when from a different vantage point he stresses that, although there are differences in personality and cultural background as well as many commonalities in the work of the three analysts (particularly in relation to the here-and-now transference), there are real differences in their basic approach. He tells us that these differences are due in some degree to their differences in *theoretical* base; i.e., the place of the oedipal conflict in the development of the child and the different forms its resolution takes in Freudian and Kleinian theory. He concludes that the work presented here is fairly representative of the work in the British Psycho-Analytical Society.

Given that psychoanalytic groups are organized around metapsychologies, we might be able to contribute to the discussion at this point by suggesting yet another factor—a narcissistic/cultural factor that helps explain group differences. As part of the introduction to this study Hill observed that psychoanalysis is unique in that it is about the very practitioners and theorists who end up supporting one version or another. Thus, the various metapsychologies are likely to attract different personalities as adherents, and the cultures of the different groups organized around these metapsychologies will reinforce different professional/personal characteristics. In addition, the style associated with each group may be based on identifications with the actual and mythic personalities and analytic styles of the charismatic leaders after whom the groups tend to be named. The stereotypes about differences in clinical styles among the groups may have varying degrees of accuracy, but to the extent to which they are accurate, metapsychology may not be the only factor explaining such differences. The group differences in clinical styles that are commonly perceived may be a function of the psychoanalytic subcultures in which analysts are immersed, of the personality characteristics that are sanctioned and promoted, and of the styles of working that go along with such characteristics.

### *Characteristics of the Patient as a Determinant of Clinical Process*

Characteristics of the patient as a factor determining how an analyst works would seem to be an obvious issue. Among the commentators, Pine, Steiner, and Parsons make note of it, but only Pine goes into detail. In an aside Pine mentions that he suspects that there were characteristics of the Kleinian analyst's patient that elicited working in the here and now.[2] He raises the issue again and in greater detail when discussing the Freudian analyst's session. These comments are par-

---

2. The Kleinian analyst added a footnote to the effect that both the characteristics of the patient and the context of the session influenced her to change from her customary way of working—in this case to intervene early in the session.

ticularly interesting when compared to those of Ellman, who addresses the same material with different perceptions and different conclusions.

For the most part Pine does not take issue with the Freudian analyst's report of how she is working and why. He describes how the Freudian analyst, in the session she presents, has done what she has indicated is her preferred way of working. That is, she has given "priority to the analysis of the 'here and now' with reconstruction in terms of the specific patient's development being used to provide a temporal dimension to the patient's insight." However, at one point he draws our attention to a comment she makes about the patient and how it may have affected the way she worked with him.

The Freudian analyst has told us that her patient has a tendency to intellectualize. Pine suggests that this tendency has caused her to orient her interventions toward "stirring the emotional pot" with the here-and-now interventions. And later, discussing the need for interventions that bring about both "experiencing" and "understanding," he draws our attention to a lengthy intervention she makes, of which he is mildly critical. Although he does not say it explicitly, there seems to be an implication that the Freudian analyst's lengthy intervention at the end of the session—an intervention leaning too much toward understanding and too little toward experiencing—may have been elicited by the patient's tendency toward intellectualization.

Pine's perceptions of this, juxtaposed against Ellman's thoughts about the same material, highlight the effects of one's response to pluralism. What for Pine was a mildly intellectualized intervention determined by a characteristic of the patient was for Ellman a moment in which metapsychology (reconstruction of the infantile neurosis) comes to bear on the process. Of course both metapsychology and the characteristic of the patient may be interacting as determinants—the traits of the patient affecting the degree to which metapsychology is drawn upon. In this session the patient's characteristic intellectualization determines the Freudian analyst's choice of working in the here and now, and occasionally, that same characteristic draws the Freudian analyst into an (overly) lengthy intervention. Indeed, it is likely that at any given moment each of the determinants of clinical process will act as a condition for the degree of influence of the others.

Pine and Ellman, who are both members of the Freudian group at NYU, are perceiving things in accordance with their responses to pluralism. Pine's emphasis on the influence of the patient fits with his universalist proposal for a multiple model based on the four psychologies of psychoanalysis. That is, at different moments an analyst should draw from among an array of models to find a mode of working that fits best—in this instance in response to patient characteristics. Ellman's perception of the Freudian analyst is in keeping with his particularist response to pluralism. From this position he argues that the Freudian analyst's Freudian roots should and do inevitably influence her technique. And again, their conclusions are not mutually exclusive. What goes on in clinical-life-as-lived is undoubtedly multiply determined.

### Context as a Determinant of Clinical Process

Pine draws our attention to the context of the sessions as a factor determining the course of an analytic session. In doing so he intersperses comments about the effects of patient characteristics. This is perhaps because context and patient characteristics have a strong interaction, and it is difficult to discuss one without referring to the other. However, it is also in keeping with the fact that multiplicity is at the heart of Pine's brand of universalism. Pine lets us know what he means by context and how it influences clinical process by contrasting the sessions presented by the Kleinian and the Independent analyst.

Pine describes the context of the Kleinian analyst's session as (1) it is the first session after a summer vacation, (2) the patient has missed the previous session, and (3) the patient has been kept waiting three minutes. Pine notes that the Kleinian analyst consistently focuses on the transference manifestations. However, he also notes that this patient is apparently one whose "associative style or general character" allows and/or encourages working in the here and now of the transference. Pine states that he cannot determine whether the fact that this session was focused on the transference was a function of the Kleinian theory to which the analyst subscribes or the personal predisposition of the Kleinian analyst. But he *can* see that the character of the patient and the events making up the context of the session did lend themselves to this style of working. He writes, "There is a very strong determinative *context* for this session: it is after a vacation and the analyst is late. It is like a session presurgery or after the death of a parent in which the analyst feels he or she knows what the content is *likely* to be about."

Pine goes on to contrast the Kleinian analyst's session, with its emphasis on the here and now, with that of the Independent analyst in which the manifest material is brought to bear on what is going on outside the session and often on what has gone on in the past. Again Pine draws our attention to the context of the session in interaction with the influence of the patient.

The context of the Independent analyst's session is termination. Pines argues that it has had a pronounced influence on technique because of particular characteristics of this patient's history and pathology. That is, it has influenced the Independent analyst to ignore largely the here and now and instead to shape his interventions in a manner that communicates, "This is what we've learned together; this is my parting gift to you." Thus, for Pine it is not that the metapsychology of the Independent group leads the Independent analyst to focus more on the past or on outside the session than on the here and now, nor that the Independent analyst's personal style emphasizes one of these modes over another. Rather, and in keeping with Pine's response to pluralism, the context—termination—has been the most pronounced determinant of clinical process in *this* session with *this* patient.

What, if anything, might we conclude from the various comments about the determinants of clinical process—about the relative effects of metapsychology, patient characteristics, analyst characteristics, and context of the session? We have attempted to show that one's response to pluralism drives the perceptions and conclusion about what is determining clinical process. Certainly there are several different parts to the elephant being examined. Obviously, to think in terms of isolated variables is to miss the forest for the trees, and we have suggested that it is likely that the interrelations among the determinants have been underappreciated. But perhaps we can go beyond that.

It is useful to employ Pine's strategy (1990) for integrating multiple points of view as we attempt to come to grips with the intricacies of clinical processes as seen from the vantages of particularist, eclectic, and universalist positions. Under different conditions any one determinant of clinical process may be more or less pronounced than the others, this may change during the course of a session and/or during the course of an analysis, and the determinants interact with one another. This provides a framework for thinking about clinical process in all its complexity. For example, these are some possibilities: (1) depending on the characteristics of an individual analyst, a metapsychology will have a more or less pronounced effect, and this, in turn, may vary depending on the charac-

teristics of the patient and on the context; (2) with some patients the characteristics of the analyst will have more influence and with others less influence; (3) in some contexts the
characteristics of the patient and of the analyst will have a diminished effect; (4) with some metapsychologies the influence
of the characteristics of the patients is more pronounced; (5)
with some analysts the characteristics of the patient will consistently have less effect than with others, and so on.

A similar degree of flexibility in thinking might be ex-
ercised concerning the debate over common ground. That
is, the question of the linkage between theory and technique
should perhaps be rephrased from whether or not they are
linked to what are the conditions determining the extent of
linkage. In addition, it might further the debate to consider
that the degree of linkage *in theory* may differ from the
degree of linkage in clinical-life-as-lived. Thus with some
analysts, and with some patients, and in some contexts
metapsychology might play a greater role than with others.
Additionally, we would add that the question of whether or
not the metapsychologies are metaphors or not might be rephrased as which aspects of the metapsychologies are metaphorical and which should be taken literally.

Finally, the study of the determinants of clinical processes points to a conclusion that can bring our speculating
to a close. That is, perhaps the therapeutic actions of psychoanalysis are sufficiently varied and the analytic process
sufficiently robust that they can tolerate the diverse ways that
we work and still maintain their integrity. Perhaps, like our
metapsychologies, we need to think of the analytic process
as sufficiently elastic to accommodate a variety of methods
and styles without losing sight of analytic goals. Mark Gehrie
(1993) puts it well: "If we mean to maintain the goal of the
fullest possible exploration of the patient's mental life, then
technical modalities become secondary to the fulfillment of
such expectations" (p. 1098).

## The Status of the Oedipal Conflict

Perhaps the most striking aspect of the responses to our attempt to assess the status of the oedipal conflict in current psychoanalytic thinking is the apparent consensus about radical change. We see this when Parsons (Chapter 10) comments that a "passing remark of the Freudian analyst shows us another theoretical shift. She says that in this session her patient was bringing oedipal material 'which had not been much in evidence in the analysis before.' And this is three years into an analysis conducted by a leading Contemporary Freudian, of all the groups in the British Society the most 'classical' in its origins." We see it again when Pine wonders "what is happening to the oedipal phase? Imagine how absent it might have been if the editors had not specifically asked for oedipal content."

If the participants in this study are representative of current thinking, then what was once accepted as *the* developmental watershed and cornerstone of clinical work is now seen as a phase among phases, a conflict among conflicts, and, perhaps, as a metaphor among metaphors. And although, as Burgner states, "We are all aware of the vital organizational value of the oedipal experience in the structuring of internal object relationships," the same could be said of rapprochement experiences, depressive experiences (see Steiner's comments in Chapter 11), mirroring and idealizing experiences, attunement experiences, and the like.

In her opening statements, the Freudian analyst writes, "The task of finding an 'oedipal' session for presentation was far from easy. Possibly this was due to my own technical approach which, although rooted in developmental thinking, gives priority to the analysis of the 'here and now.'" She goes on to write, "For me the awareness of the tremendous importance of preoedipal factors also contributed to the difficulty in finding an oedipal session. . . ."

Pine provides a more general explanation for why although "the oedipal phase and oedipal fantasy and wishes are very much present . . . they are not the full story and often not the main story." He posits that our conception of it has changed due to a more sophisticated understanding of development, an expansion of theory, and perhaps because of a change in the zeitgeist (postmodern uncertainty) that allows us to "listen more openly and hear things in more diverse ways."

The same might be said for the thinking about the relationship between preoedipal and oedipal material. Thinking in terms of "either–or" has been replaced by a more complex view of mental life positing "and." There is apparent consensus that the preoedipal and oedipal aspects of mental life are inevitably and perhaps inextricably intertwined. The Freudian analyst states that "preoedipal factors inevitably color oedipal conflicts, which we seldom see in pure culture." Regarding the Kleinian and the Independent analysts' patients, Pine, Ellman, and Burgner all note that, although the situations are triangular, the dyadic dynamics are more pronounced. Finally, Parsons writes, "All three presentations thus confirm that oedipal and preoedipal aspects of psychopathology are indissoluble and that any clinical material is bound to contain an expression of both."

All this seems to suggest that there are varying degrees of oedipal resolution and varying degrees of preoedipal influence. Parsons takes us to the next step: "We must not expect to analyze one separately from the other. How, then, to avoid chaos as we are confronted with a complexity that needs disentangling, but must not be falsely simplified?"

The only point of controversy that emerges is the enduring difference in Kleinian and Freudian theorizing about the timing of oedipal developments, and even this may boil down to a semantic dispute when it comes to clinical work.

Steiner articulates the conceptual difference between Kleinians and Freudians.

> Melanie Klein recognized early stages of the Oedipus complex beginning soon after birth and becoming well established by the onset of the depressive position in the first half of the first year. Kleinian analysts might discern primitive versions of the oedipal configuration in various aspects of the case material presented, particularly when a triangular configuration was present. A Contemporary Freudian analyst would be more inclined to consider oedipal phantasies to arise later between the third and fifth year of life and to conceptualize it in terms of more mature whole object relationships. . . . She does not consider everything triangular to be oedipal, and it is this conceptualization that leads her to place more emphasis on the more mature elements of the Oedipus complex that her patient illustrated so nicely.

Ellman focuses on the fact that the Kleinian and the Independent analysts have chosen sessions in which they believed they were dealing with oedipal phenomena but that he (a Freudian) does not conceptualize the patients as having arrived at the oedipal level nor does he think that the analysts have addressed material as if it is oedipal.

Ellman (Chapter 6) argues that the sessions are filled with preoedipal material and, moreover, that the Kleinian analyst and the Independent analyst deal with it as preoedipal material. He makes the point, as does the Freudian analyst in her introduction, that "triangulation does not necessarily imply oedipal dynamics or structure. The capacity for object love . . . is a necessary concomitant of oedipal dynamics, despite the fact that this developed faculty may be severely hampered by intrapsychic conflict." He sees the fact that the Independent and Kleinian analysts have chosen these sessions as representative for this project as indicative of the terminological confusion that plagues the field—that we use the same terms to mean different things: "[I]t may be that what we called oedipal dynamics is a result of a different semantic code rather than a difference in our understanding of the case material."

According to Ellman the issue of whether or not the patient has arrived at an oedipal level of development is important because in the case of a narcissistic patient one would expect and use the analytic process to be the central mutative factor in the therapy rather than interpretation. He make this point in his assessment of the Independent analyst's presentation in which, Ellman argues, a holding environment has been the prominent mutative factor during the course of the treatment. If Ellman speaks as a Freudian, then his comment is a good example of how the term *Freudian* no longer means what it used to (interpretation is not *the* mutative factor). From the point of view of furthering the field it is keeping with Parsons' call for the next stage of development. That is, if there is now consensus that preoedipal and oedipal issues are indissoluble, the question becomes how to work with the complexity of their intertwinement.

### Conceptual Schemes for Assessing Clinical Process

Conducting this type of study confronts one with the problems of systematically comparing and contrasting the various theoretical orientations, that is, with problems of format and instructions to the authors and commentators, with delimitations on the focus of each, and with establishing ways of evaluating the wealth of data that accumulate. We attempted to impose as much structure as possible. In order to keep the focus limited and to have something concrete to evaluate, we instructed the authors to discuss a single session that had the same central issue: "an oedipal session." We also asked for a "regular session, warts and all" in the attempt to get a picture of clinical-life-as-lived. We were not interested in idealized sessions, sessions that were particularly good, or sessions that were particularly dramatic. We instructed the commentators to compare and contrast the sessions presented and to avoid any kind of supervision or second guessing—a process that we have found to be unproductive. Finally, whereas the authors were focused primarily on their patients and the commentators focused primarily on the sessions presented, we limited our focus to the commentary (of the authors and/or the commentators) for our summary. To our surprise and pleasure there was a fortuitous byproduct of the project that we believe will be useful for future projects like this or any attempt to ascertain what is going on in clinical-life-as-lived, i.e., conceptual schemes for thinking about clinical process.

### A Differentiation of the Work in the Here and Now of the Transference

Pine draws our attention to the vagueness of the concept of here and now and differentiates three kinds of working in the here and now. First there is working "from the outside into the office. 'You think you are talking about something out there, but it is really about me (or about us)'—this in contrast to Freud's earliest discovery about transference which goes: 'What you think you are feeling or imagining about me is really about person X from your past.'"

In another form of working in the here-and-now, the "transference is worked with because it is brought in by some patients who often, or even regularly, come in and talk about the analyst and their relation to him or her. The analyst works with this here and now presumably with the underlying idea that the analytic events are a microcosm of the patient's world, and that therefore the work is properly done within the analysis."

Finally, a third form of working with the here and now of the transference "refers to enactments: 'It's not what you are saying here that counts (at this moment) because what's really important is what is happening between us, a something that you are living out—in your mood, your way of speaking, the atmosphere you set up, the way you entrap me into being, and the like.'"

Pine's criticism of the term "working in the here-and-now" as meaning too many things and his laying out several different kinds of that work are surely applicable to other technical terms that we take for granted but that on closer examination are probably a source of confusion and misunderstanding among analysts. There are perhaps other forms of working in the here-and-now, and there are undoubtedly other technical terms that need to be clarified. Each is commonly used with the idea that we all are doing the same thing when we do them, but each can take on several forms and when comparing and contrasting sessions of different analysts and different patients it is important to be specific about how they are carried out.

### The Tempo of the Work

All of the commentators have drawn our attention to what Parsons has called "the tempo of the work"—the Kleinian analyst's session having the quicker tempo in contrast to the Freudian analyst's and the Independent analyst's more moderate pace. The Kleinian analyst seems to lean forward into the work, whereas the Freudian and the Independent analysts sit back. Theoretical orientation and the characters of the analysts and the patients have been looked to for explanation of the variations in this parameter. Parsons provides us with a scheme for articulating and appreciating tempo as an important factor in clinical process that has varying uses and that should be attended to in that it involves the stance of the analyst and the aim of the work. It can serve as a model for schemes that provide an unbiased appreciation of the complexity of clinical process and of different approaches.

For Parsons the different tempos are more than simple differences in personal style. Rather, tempo indicates "a different attitude to the transference between the two analysts." The Kleinian analyst is keeping up moment to moment with the "shifts in the transference, so that the most fleeting of affects or fantasies may be caught on the wing and interpreted. What it does not emphasize so much, however, is the slower, longer-term, consistent evolution of the transference in a certain direction." By contrast the Freudian analyst "is using the transference in a different way: not to offer a series of particular insights but cumulatively to arrive at understanding an experience that only develops itself fully over the length of the session."

Parsons sees the tempo as a variable for coming to grips with the complexity of material. The Freudian analyst prefer(s) to "watch and wait to understand, while an evolving process gradually allows clarity to appear so that the complexity becomes interpretable." The Kleinian analyst, alternatively, seems to work out of a conviction "that the elements making up the complexity have to be grasped and examined actively before any interpreting can be done." He goes on to say that the Kleinian's style

> is a much more interventionist style of analysis, and the rhythm of the analyst's responsiveness is quite different from the Freudian's. The advantages and disadvantages of these ways of analyzing are often

discussed, and certain familiar arguments are put forward regularly. Those closer to the viewpoint of the Freudian analyst want the analyst not to be overcertain, not to tell patients what is in their minds, to wait for the nuances of the patients' state of mind to declare themselves, not to be in a hurry to understand. The concept of "negative capability" is bound to get mentioned. Those closer to the style of the Kleinian analyst may say that patients can only face their conflicts if we take up directly the anxiety that stops them from doing so, that the patient needs to see that the analyst is not afraid of the patient's feelings, and that what frightens the patient most and which she cannot confront without help is what most needs bringing into the open, so that we should not wait too long before intervening.

We might add a note to Parsons's insightful contribution. Although the tempo of the work has been discussed in terms of qualitative differences, it is perhaps best conceptualized as a continuum (the rate of analyst activity) associated with a variety of possibilities and dangers. This would allow a discussion of the effects of differing tempos across a range of possibilities and the conditions in which different tempos are called for. It is likely that some analysts, regardless of the metapsychology to which they subscribe, maintain the same tempo across patients, that the cultures associated with the various theories encourage more reticent or bolder tempos, and that these different ways of dealing with the complexity of the material will suit different analysts and different patients in varying degrees. But in the best of all analytic worlds, would it not seem obvious that the tempo should be adjusted according to the characteristics of the patient and the shifting aims of the work.

### *The Locus of the Work with the Transference*

Closely related to the tempo of the work is another parameter for which Parsons has provided another scheme for
assessing clinical process. It might be called the locus of the
work with the transference, and Parsons has found two such
sites. That is, he establishes that the Kleinian analyst is interested in bringing out and interpreting the internal object
relationships of her patient. Toward this end she illuminates
and interprets the inner world qua inner world. Oedipal
conflicts are pointed out as they are found *there.* For the
Freudian analyst and the Independent analyst the locus of
the work is between the inner and external world. The transference is treated in "a shared space *between* patient and analyst" and "the interpretative work happens *between* the patient
and the analyst." Interweaving his observations of both the
tempo and location, Parsons attributes the differences to
one's theoretical orientation.

> I have been pointing to something that is a distinc-
> tively Kleinian way of working: the evenly continu-
> ing use of a fluctuating transference to allow the
> analyst to direct interpretations to the patient's
> fantasy world of internal object relationships. The
> Freudian analyst, in contrast, shows the evolving
> use of a more progressively developing transfer-
> ence to allow interpretations of what is happening,
> both in fantasy and reality, in an analytic space that
> is shared between patient and analyst.

Singling out the issue of locus, the point would seem to be
that each of the analysts has his or her preferred spot in which
to work—directly on the inner world known to the analyst
through the transference (Modern Kleinian) or directly on

the transference interpreted as a reflection of the inner world (Contemporary Freudian and Independent).

Finally, Parsons emphasizes a larger point that he makes throughout his commentary, i.e., the differences among the groups is largely a matter of emphasis. He notes that "the Freudian analyst does of course, interpret the patient's fantasies; an inner world of the patient is certainly being elucidated." And he points out that the Independent analyst's work with the transference is in relation to the "historical events in the family . . . together with the fantasies and the anxieties attached to them in the child's and his parents' minds at the time." Thus, concerning the locus of the work with the transference—directly in the inner world, on the space between the inner and external worlds created by the analysis as a reflection of the inner world, and in that shared space in relationship to the patient's history—he concludes that "all three analysts use all three of these approaches. They are interrelated strands in the work of analysis that cannot be separated from each other. *Our three presentations show us, nonetheless, the difference of emphasis that different analysts may put on one approach or another*" (italics added).

We might again add a note to Parsons' observations. In this case it adds yet another determinant to our list of those affecting clinical process. That is, the gender differences among the analytic dyads. The Freudian analyst and the Independent analyst are conducting cross-gender analyses. The Kleinian analyst has a same-gender analysis. Looking at the preferred locus of the work with the transference through the lens of gender raises several questions. Are women more comfortable going into one another's inner worlds? If so, does the Freudian analyst respect her male patient's needs for a measure of distance and therefore conducts a more "distant" analysis to avoid eliciting an experience of intrusiveness? And does the Independent analyst conduct an analysis tempered by his gender-determined need for working in a transitional space rather than directly in the patient's inner world? And, finally, do the Kleinian analyst and her female patient create a more purely feminine analysis?

## Conclusion

We have attempted to summarize and integrate the commentary on process notes presented by training analysts from Contemporary Freudian, Modern Kleinian, and Independent orientations at the British Psycho-Analytical Society. Occasionally we attempted a synthesis or added notes of our own. We have also attempted to illuminate and demonstrate how pluralism is a positive driving force in psychoanalysis. Perhaps the best indication of that possibility has been the fruits of this effort. Key to the effort was the collection of dedicated and talented analysts making up the working group. Our thanks goes to them.

Finally, it is our hope that this study will engender others like it. The conceptual schemes for assessing clinical process are meant to help those efforts. And although small samples have obvious limitations, over time, like the dots on a photograph, they evolve into a full picture from which we can draw conclusions. Thus far, this method of studying the psychoanalytic situation is the best we have come up with in a discipline that does not lend itself to traditional empirical methods. Depending on how it is approached, pluralism is both a fragmentation of the field and a motor of developing convergences. Most institutes find themselves caught up in the conflict of conservative and progressive forces. Cross-theoretical studies bend the dynamics toward the latter.

# References

Etchegoyen, H. (1991). *The Fundamentals of Psychoanalytic Technique.* London: Karnac.

Gehrie, M. J. (1993). Psychoanalytic technique and the capacity to reflect. *Journal of the American Psychoanalytic Association* 41:1083–1111.

Greenberg, J. R., and Mitchell, S. (1983). *Object Relations in Psychoanalytic Theory.* Cambridge: Harvard University Press.

Joseph, B. (1988). Object relations in clinical practice. *Psychoanalytic Quarterly* 57:626–642.

King, P., and Steiner, R., eds. (1991). *The Freud-Klein Controversies, 1941–45.* London: Tavistock/Routledge.

Levine, H. (1992). Freudian and Kleinian theory. *Journal of the American Psychoanalytic Association* 40:801–826.

Modell, A. (1994). Common ground or divided ground. *Psychoanalytic Inquiry* 14:201–211.

Pine, F. (1990). *Drive, Ego, Object and Self.* New York: Basic Books.

Racker, H. (1968). *Transference and Countertransference.* London: Hogarth.

Richards, A. D., and Richards, A. K. (in press). Notes on psychoanalytic theory and its consequences for technique. *Journal of Clinical Psychoanalysis.*

Sandler, J., and Sandler, A.-M. (1994). The past unconscious, the present unconscious, and interpretation of the transference. *Psychoanalytic Inquiry* 4:367–399.

Schafer, R. (1990). The search for common ground. *International Journal of Psycho-Analysis* 71:49–52.

Wallerstein, R. S. (1990). Psychoanalysis: the common ground. *International Journal of Psycho-Analysis* 71:3–20.

—— (1992). *The Common Ground of Psychoanalysis.* Northvale, NJ: Jason Aronson.

# Index